THE RED-LIGHT THERAPY:

RED-LIGHT FOR YOUR OWN PERSONAL HEALTH. ANTIAGING METHOD FOR YOUR SKINCARE, WEIGHT LOSS, HAIR LOSS, AND ACNE.

A SELF-HELP GUIDE……

Samantha Clooney

Table of Contents

in this book.

By reading this document, the reader agrees that under no circumstances is the author responsible for any losses, direct or indirect, incurred due to the use of the information contained within this document, including, but not limited to, errors, omissions, or inaccuracies.

Introduction

Red-light Therapy systems are starting to become more popular, but before they develop themselves, it seems that there could be an excellent way to go. It appears to be a bit high-tech and sci-fi for many people, while it is considered just a modern trend for others.

The picture of red-light therapy tools of high-tech space ages can be well justified due to their existence.

First, NASA developed them to cultivate plant life in space, attempting to replicate the sun's effectiveness. Eventually, it was found that the light had beneficial and restoratory effects on the skin of the astronauts, so the focus of the research went on.

The technology made its earthly debut as a test therapy for cancer patients, and the reports made available showed that this promise was shown.

As further review and evaluation, the fundamental understanding of the consequences and the advantages of the red-light was understood. The red light penetrates underneath the skin and facilitates cellular rejuvenation and collagen production.

Both these behaviors decline as we get older. Therefore, our body begins to show signs and symptoms of aging when red light promotes cell rejuvenation to a younger person, why plumps are decreased, and pores are reduced.

It also destroys germs under the skin layers, becoming a popular technique for clearing adult and cyst acne patients. The red light is also adequate at a bone tissue and muscle level with similar rejuvenation benefits, thanks to its actual permeation depth.

Muscle groups and general weight losses usually decrease quickly, pain is relieved, and pain is provided for disorders such as arthritis.

After the clinical studies have been completed, the devices have started appearing in specialist saloons and skin therapy centers before finally reaching the consumer market and ending their journey from the open area to the canapé.

These products are by no means overnight treatments, they need dedication and time like most treatments for work, and their impact differs from person to person. However, they are one of the most prospective developments in the anti-aging and pain relief industry for an extended period.

Beauty is a significant part of their personality for many women. So the aging aspect apprehends many people. Such women try to revitalize their skin and make it look young again, but they do not do so to most of their degree.

However, recent research has confirmed that a particular type of treatment will revitalize the skin tissues and reappear young and vibrant. It is known as the Rejuve anti-aging method. This new idea in skin rejuvenation utilizes the groundbreaking Red-light

Therapy to reverse the skin's effects of aging, dry skin, and wrinkles.

In general, skin creams and skin ointments with anti-aging effects do not positively alter the patient's skin as they focus mainly on the outside of the skin.

It means that the cream's primary purpose is to purify the pores and to try to make the skin glow in a just tone. Though, without adequately revitalizing the inner tissues, the chances of turning the clock back on your skin are much smaller.

The use of this special therapy has been highly encouraging. Studies have found that the red light penetrates the skin and induce an improvement in your skin by enhancing the production of collagen, which is your body's most essential protein needed for the repair and/or replacement of weakened and broken tissues.

The question in most people's minds now is whether or not this particular type of therapy is safe? This special type of therapy procedure is almost the same as tanning, with only a small change. A specific type of therapy can either be used in a rehabilitation stand or a bed.

This unique type of treatment is quite simple, and it's a perfect way to turn the clock back and look young again.

Let's get started

Chapter 1: What is Red-light Therapy?

Red-light therapy, also recognized as photobiomodulation or low-level laser therapy (LLLT), has increasingly become a standard type of treatment in the areas of neurology, physiotherapy, and dermatology. More specifically, the use of red light-emitting diodes (LEDs) managed to reach through a person's skin has shown considerable possibilities for cell growth, tissue repair, and pain management. It is also active in improving the health of the joints and muscles, increasing the side effects of cancer treatment, and adding to aging and hair loss symptoms. LLLT can be used to treat depression, improve your mood and help you feel less stressed. Light therapy is one of the earliest therapeutic modalities known. Romans first used sun therapy, and solar treatment was also studied by ancient Greeks, Chinese, and Indians.

There is no doubt that light has biological effects: the body needs sunlight to be safe in reality. Clinical studies are now investigating how various wavelengths of light affect the body at the cellular level, the diseases that can be successfully treated by light therapy, and the optimum circumstances required to receive the effects of light-based care.

LED is a light-emitting diode. "This operates by transmitting infrared lights (causing heat) of various wavelengths/spectrums that have different skin-care benefits." "The illumination of amber activates collagen and elastin. Red-light is most widely used to promote movement. White light penetrates most and tends to close down and reduce inflammation. Blue light is destroying microbes. "Systems relay light waves deep into the skin through LED therapy to induce natural intracellular responses. Depending on the light, the skin may respond differently." When[color] red, your skin will respond by developing, expanding, and improving the cellular structure. Red light is also believed to impact oil glands to reduce cytokines that cause inflammations and play an important role in chronic acne. In the case of blue light, different wavelengths promote the development of oxygen radicals that destroy acne bacteria, all without affecting the body, "

What Is Red-light Therapy?

Red-light therapy (RLT) is a standard medical procedure that uses low-level red-light rays to address skin problems such as lines, bruises, or chronic injuries, among other factors.

In the early 1990s, RLT was used by researchers to help grow space-based crops. Scientists have found that intense light from red light-emitting diodes (LEDs) has led to the development and photosynthesis of plant cells.

The red light was then researched for its possible use in medicine, more precisely to figure out whether RLT can raise energy within human cells. The researchers hoped RLT could efficiently treat muscle atrophy, slow wound healing, and bone density problems caused by weightlessness during space travel.

Red-light therapy is a therapeutic technique that utilizes red-tinted illumination to activate the body's natural defense systems and provide relief from various diseases. It gives quick results for people with a variety of skin problems.

Red-light therapy uses heat and intense illumination to promote circulation, increase collagen production, and improve the skin's natural healing capacity.

It is non-invasive and does not produce ultraviolet rays. Infrared beams reach skin tissue to a thickness of up to 10 millimeters. This extra energy allows skin cells to increase the production of fresh collagen and the recycling of collagen and elastin fibers—critical components of skin regeneration.

Red-light acne therapy helps teenagers with skin problems by helping to eliminate clogged pores. Facial red-light treatment helps in the production of nervous tics. Just as natural sunlight assists with mild depression, red-light therapy can boost moods and increase stress in the winter months. If that wasn't enough, there are even reports that the activation of ATP in the body can assist with different forms of sexual arousal in both men and women.

Types Of Red-light Therapy Devices

Having a system will be the next logical step if you are well educated about red-light therapy and want to take advantage of its many benefits. The secret to choosing the' correct' one will rely on a variety of factors-specifically, the illness that you want to handle. Understandably, most people will choose to consult a doctor or dermatologist to ensure that they are not only correctly handled with a licensed red-light therapy tool but have also been approved by the FDA. And, because most insurance companies still do not provide regular long-term LLLT sessions, medical treatment can become quite expensive even in a medical condition. Most spas, fitness centers, or tanning lounges still provide red-light therapy. Still, because daily appointments will be of the most significant benefit, services at these facilities can also be included.

Below is a list of Red-light Therapy Devices:

- Handheld
- Beds
- Tabletop lamps
- Masks (face only)
- Box-light
- Free-standing lamps
- Helmet (hair growth)

- Flex pads- (for back, legs, knees, arms)
- Screens
- Laser comb

Know What To Look For In A Red-light Therapy Device:

With a wide range of product models to choose from, you'll want to know what to look for before you make a purchase. They should be mindful that many red-light therapy systems (depending on the length of the session) will use a great deal of energy—even more so if they choose the wrong machine. Doing some homework on the design and technical aspects of the products you are interested in and reviewing consumer reports and feedback can help you make an informed decision.

Because different devices come with varying energy rates. It will be necessary to use one with the appropriate wavelength and energy intensity to ensure that the light will penetrate the skin around 8-10 nm. You should also be mindful that certain parts of the body must consume just as much energy for the light to be efficient. Of starters, different conditions, such as joint pain, can require more extended, more intense sessions when managing acne on your body and may need shorter sessions with less severity.

Wavelengths: Most apps provide a similar array of wavelengths- and each spectrum will have its advantages. Generally speaking, at-home devices are between 600 nm and 800 nm, but you can find ones up to 900 nm in the near-infrared zone. The mid-600 nm level to the low-to mid-800 nm range is optimal, according to scientific research, and can be highly effective for several conditions.

Power production: The system's energy output would depend on joules, the default power unit provided to your cells during therapy. It will be essential to determine how much energy your system absorbs, as cells can only consume a certain amount to be successful. Subsequently, the excess energy (to some extent) can be toxic to the cells.

Switch period for sessions: another factor will be its time to transmit heat to your body. How long does it take for the fuel to enter the' targeted' areas of the body? How long will it take to get the correct amount of energy to the environment without placing the cells at risk? Sometimes, LLLT tools will include the required information to help you quantify energy output in joules per minute-some will even provide a table/chart to make it easier for the user.

Understanding Red-light Wavelengths

The light is moving along a continuum of wavelengths. Red or infrared-light dropping within the wavelength range of 650-850 nm is highly beneficial and often referred to as a "therapeutic window." Such wavelengths of light are bioactive to humans and influence the activity of our cells.

Red-light absorbs wavelengths from 620-700 nm. Both red wavelengths are active and provide health benefits, although some wavelengths are more efficient than others-especially those between 630-680 nm. Visible red light within this spectrum may penetrate deep into the body, producing rejuvenating and calming effects for various health conditions.

Sunlight contains an element of red light; this light spectrum leads to the improved feeling of well-being that we feel after a few hours outdoors. Red-light therapy products, such as those sold by PlatinumLED Therapy Lights, channel regenerative red-light wavelengths with no more harmful UVA or UVB light rays that can cause skin cancer or premature aging.

How does Red-light Therapy works?

It is believed that red-light functions by generating a biochemical cell reaction that activates mitochondria. Mitochondria is the cell's powerhouse— where the cell's energy is produced. Adenosine triphosphate (ATP) is the energy-carrying molecule found in the cells of all living things.

A cell can generate more ATP through the work of mitochondria with RLT. Cells can work more efficiently with more energy, rejuvenate themselves, and repair damage.

RLT is distinct from the laser and intense pulsed light (IPL) treatment because it does not harm the skin's surface. Laser and pulsed light therapy work by causing programmed damage to the skin's outer layer, resulting in tissue repair. By actively inducing skin regeneration, RLT bypasses this problematic step. The RLT light penetrates about 5 millimeters below the skin's surface.

What is Red-light Therapy used for?

Since the original space studies, many clinical trials and dozens of experimental tests have been conducted to determine whether RLT has health benefits. There have been positive findings from several problems, but the effects of red-light therapy remain a source of conflict. For example, the Medicare and Medicaid Services Centers (CMS) have concluded insufficient evidence to show that these innovations are safer for wounds, ulcers, and pain than traditional medicines.

Additional clinical research is needed to confirm that RLT is effective. At the moment, moreover, there is some evidence to suggest that RLT may have the following benefits:

- Facilitates wound regeneration and tissue repair
- Enhances hair growth of people with androgen alopecia
- Assist in the short-term diagnosis of carpal tunnel syndrome
- Encourages healing of slow-healing wounds, such as diabetic foot ulcers
- Decreases psoriasis lesions
- helps in short-term relaxation of discomfort and daily weakness in people with rheumatoid arthritis

- Reduces many of the side effects of cancer treatment, including oral mucositis

- Enhances skin tone and develops collagen

- helps to eliminate wrinkles while helping to mitigate sun harm

- Affirmatively avoids persistent cold sores from herpes

- Improves degenerative knees osteoarthritis.

- Helps prevent scarring

- Relieves pain and inflammation for people suffering from the Achilles tendons.

Understanding How Red-light Therapy Works

Therefore, red-light therapy is the therapeutic practice of using red and ultraviolet light rays to help manage health conditions and encourage general well-being. You may also have referred to other terms as red-light care, such as:

- Low-level light therapy (LLLT)

- Photobiomodulation (PBM)

- Soft laser therapy

- Biostimulation

- Photonic stimulation

- Low-power laser therapy

- Cold laser therapy

Chromophores in our cell mitochondria absorb and transform red and infrared-light photons into energy during the treatment of red light. Mitochondria are the powerhouse of the cells. It produces an energy molecule known as "adenosine triphosphate" (ATP), fueling other cellular processes.

Once the body has absorbed this red-light power, the cells build new proteins such as collagen and elastin and rebuild the cells. Red light provides the cells a helping hand, ensuring the mitochondria meet their capacity and supplying it with a full fuel tank, which results in optimal performance for the organism.

You can equate the cycle to photosynthesis, where plants consume sunlight and turn it into complex molecules. In the case of red-light therapy, they consume the power of red-light photons to increase our neuronal capacity, facilitate the use of oxygen within the cell, and produce ATP or cellular gas.

There is nothing magical or new-age about it - the mechanism by which red-light changes body tissue at the cellular level has been scientifically proven. Improving the efficiency of mitochondria in the body increases the overall performance and health of the organ.

Understanding Near Infrared (NIR) Light Wavelengths

Thus visible red-light is one-quarter of red-light therapy; near-infrared-light (NIR) is the other half. Near-infrared radiation (NIR) lies just above the visible light spectrum, with wavelengths varying from 700 nm to more than 1,100 nm. Compared to red light, not all wavelengths within this spectrum are similarly effective in healing: wavelengths from 800-880 nm appear to offer the most significant therapeutic benefit.

The body absorbs NIR light in the same manner as visible red light by chromophores in our cells. Upon ingestion, several biochemical healing pathways are activated, facilitating recovery and regeneration. Nevertheless, there is a big difference between red and near-infrared light: near-infrared light can penetrate more into the tissue of the body due to shorter wavelengths. Red-light therapy systems that blend both red-light and near-infrared-light provide good curing power as they provide a variety of clinical wavelengths. Such wavelengths can be aimed at a variety of issues. For example, red-light wavelength hs may penetrate deep into the skin, facilitating collagen production and healing wounds. In contrast, near-infrared light may penetrate deeper into the body's tissue to effectively reach deep injuries, muscles, and joint pain.

Both Platinum LED light therapy systems are accessible in either a red 660 nm or near-infrared 850 m illumination for optimum therapeutic benefits.

How Does Red-light Therapy Help Mitigate The Effects Of Stress, Illness, Or Injury?

When we are sick, depressed, and wounded, the potential of cell mitochondria to work at total capacity is compromised. In the rapidly-paced, pressure-saturated sense of the natural world, many of us are inconveniently aware of the impact of increased tension on our skin— restless nights and strict deadlines cause us to look tacky out, haggard, and older than our actual age. Cosmetic remedies can only provide temporary treatment to what is an issue within our bodies. When we are anxious and sick, mitochondria begin to produce more nitric oxide. Nitric oxide is harmful because it interferes with the absorption of oxygen within the cell, induces oxidative stress, and eventually inhibits the output of ATP, the cell's fuel source. As a consequence, the cell could die.

Red or near-infrared light (delivered within acceptable wavelengths and energy levels) shields the cell from harm induced by nitric oxide. The destructive ability of nitric oxide is reduced by removing red-light photons, enabling the cell to proceed successfully, consuming oxygen and producing ATP. Only red-light therapy may enter the cell's mitochondria to promote healing and growth, enhance health, efficiency, and general well-being.

The Depth Of Penetration Of Red-light

Red or infrared light can penetrate deeper into the skin than nearly any other light wavelength.

When described above, infrared light has a range of penetration that exceeds specific wavelengths of light, which means it can penetrate the body's underlying tissues below the surface. This deep tissue penetration also leads to light therapy, which causes a systemic and physiological effect on the whole body rather than a focused impact on a particular area. Red-light can penetrate to a depth of 5-10 mm under optimal conditions. LED lamps (light-emitting diode) used in Platinum Light Therapy provide the most dynamic red and infrared light ranges for optimum absorption. Modern light bulbs such as halogen and incandescent do not emit sufficient light to regenerate and repair cells.

Red-light Energy Output: Why Platinum LED Therapy Lights Are Superior

Although red-light wavelengths manipulate the effectiveness of the treatment, several people don't realize that the energy output of the red-light therapy device is just as critically important. Currently, VAST varies between LED red-light therapy devices on the market. Many emit an extremely low energy output, even though they consume a lot of power.

Platinum LED Therapy Lights was the first LED Red-light Therapy company to bring the energy calculation idea to the table. After years of experience in manufacturing LED lights to promote plant growth, it made sense for us to calculate the light's energy output, which had a substantial impact on its effectiveness. The emissions of our horticultural lighting are measured in terms of Photosynthetic Active Radiation, more informally referred to as PAR. It tests the energy strength of the LED's light growth.

The production of the LED therapy light is defined as irradiance (the radiant energy flux per unit area) and is measured in terms of MW / cm2. Over several years, they have helped inform our audience about the discrepancies between LED light manufacturers concerning these outputs. The energy output of the Platinum LED Therapy lighting is maximized to ensure the therapy of red-light is done safely. The lamps produce more irradiance than any other LED light currently on the market.

Just Platinum LED Therapy Lights can provide greater red-light or near-infrared-light penetration than any other light is capable of achieving.

Chapter 2: How Does Red-light Therapy Work?

What can Red-light Therapy do for your skin?

NASA discovered that red and infrared LEDs (light-emitting diodes) healed injuries faster when conducting outer space plant growth tests. Light has been harnessed and studied since these discoveries, revealing countless benefits and therapeutic uses.

You will find red-light therapy in dermatology offices, chiropractor offices, doctors, spas, clinics, salons, and at home. As this therapy gains popularity, some may be skeptical, asking if this therapy works.

The straight answer is a resounding yes!

How works light therapy?

Light-emitting diodes or LED makes lengths of wave in nanometers. The bigger the number of nanometers, the lengthier the wavelength is.

• Circulation is being boosted

• Rise in collagen

• Encouraging healing and reparative processes to engage

• Increasing endorphin production

• Blocking pain transmitting neurons

As these reactions begin to occur in cells and tissues, changes occur within cells and tissues.

Hair benefits include:

• Reduced lines and wrinkles

• Diminished crow's feet

• Diminished age spots and scarring

• Smoother texture

• Smaller pores

• Tighter and firmer hair

• Brighter complexion

 • Improved collagen and elastin production

• Reduced redness

• Rosacea help

• Accelerated healing of blemishes

• Reduced inflammation

Skin benefits include:

• Pain relief.

Yellow LEDs at 590 + nanometers, red LEDs at 625-660 nanometers, and infrared LEDs at 830 + nanometers can penetrate all layers of skin where they heal and repair past damage.

When it comes to pain relief, red LEDs at 660 + nanometers and infrared LEDs at 880 + nanometers can penetrate up to 2 inches into skin, tissue, joints, and bones, relieving pain and healing.

Red-light treatment is a complex approach to skin recovery and acute and chronic pain control. It's a secure, reliable, drug-free, and robust alternative to handle a vast array of issues.

Which Home Systems have shown accurate results?

Best for Skin Rejuvenation:

DPL Therapy System-This is a hands-free, two-panel system with 660 nm red LEDs and 880 nanometer infrared LEDs.

Quasar MD-This potent handheld device uses 5 mm LEDs with 4 wavelengths at 640 nm, 660 nm, 880 nm, and 940 nm.

Baby Quasar PLUS — This handheld unit is smaller than the Quasar MD and uses 3 mm LEDs at 640 nm, 660 nm, 880 nm, and 940 nm.

ReVive Light Therapy Beauty Kit-This particular handheld device includes two eyes, one using 625 nm red and 830 nm infrared. The other head has 415-nanometer blue LEDs designed to kill acne bacteria, P. acnes.

Caribbean Sun Skin Rejuvenation Light — Another hands-free panel system that uses red LEDs at 660 nm and yellow LEDs at 590 nm Best pain systems:

DPL Therapy System — This hands-free two-panel system is not only beneficial for skin rejuvenation but also includes LEDs that help relieve pain and promote healing. The panels are removable and can be attached to body parts.

ReVive Pain Relief Light Therapy- This handheld system contains 660-nanometer red LEDs and 880-nanometer infrared LEDs.

Dpl Flex is a lightweight belt device comprising small panels inserted into pockets. Because it's versatile, it's easier to place it in more body places. Each panel contains 660 nm red LEDs and 880 nm infrared LEDs

How Red-light Therapy Can Make You Look Younger

If you read this chapter, you probably have some excellent chances of hearing red-light therapy and wondering, first, what's it in the world and secondly, what are its benefits and how will they affect you?

Red-light therapy is increasing in popularity worldwide exponentially. It has now been found in skin treatment clinics, dermatology offices, plastic surgeon offices, spas, resorts, offices, homes, and even tanning rooms.

But why is the tremendous uproar, and why is this seemingly unpretentious technology like wildfire? It is a non-invasive, pain-free, and drug-free choice that significantly benefits the skin and the entire body and well-being.

NASA found that red and infrared LEDs (light diodes) were highly beneficial to plants and significantly accelerated the healing of lesions that astronauts suffered in outer space during plant growth experiments.

Since these observations, countless studies were conducted using specific wavelengths that showed many positive results and advantages.

These studies have shown that wavelengths in the yellow, amber, red and infrared ranges penetrate deeply into every layer of the skin and give many different benefits such as:

- Collagen stimulation and Elastin production
- Redness reducing redness
- Skin reduction lines and wrinkles

The repair and healing properties within the wavelengths provide a natural way to speed up healing and alleviate pain. Red and Infrared-light therapy helps to reduce inflammation, improve endorphin production, and neural transmission block pain Increase circulation

Increased cellular energy (ATP)

Cellular damage repair To see significant results with red-light therapy, continuity, and daily treatments are necessary. It's not a treatment you can do every time and expect impressive results.

These powerful yet reassuring treatments must be performed regularly to repair and heal the skin and body. Red-light therapy provides a safe, drug-free, non-invasive, non-ablative, and supportive alternative to strengthen skin, promote healing and relieve pain effectively.

Red-light therapy is a technology that excites a small amount of magic in your skin by prompting more than 24 positive cellular responses. Red, yellow, and LEDs are designed to encourage a youthful and healthier look. Each LED color can penetrate deeper into the skin and tissues with red and infrared than the yellow LEDs.

Yellow LEDs treat sunburns, rosacea, and eczema effectively. These LEDs reduce redness and swelling while rejuvenating the skin. Several studies have shown that yellow light therapy also improves lines and wrinkles. Red and yellow LEDs are paired with the Caribbean Sun Light to encourage better, more vivid tinting.

Red LEDs stimulate the development of collagen, improve cell repair and increase circulation. Due to the high blood and water content in your tissue, your skin can readily absorb red light, which causes intense skin rejuvenation and cell regeneration.

Red-light therapy helps lower lines and wrinkles, decrease age, decrease the scar, promote a more even skin sound, and more.

Naked in the human eye, infrared LEDs reach deeper through skin and tissue than red and yellow LEDs, countering aging signs by rapid healing and refilling dermal and epidermal cells and activating repair procedures. The DPL Therapy System incorporates red and infrared LEDs into one hand-free unit that encourages younger-looking skin with fewer lines and wrinkles.

As we age, our production of collagen and elastin slows down, and cell turnover decreases. Free radicals and severity will hurt your skin, which will make it look aged and dead.

Red-light therapy has shown that the symptoms of aging are reversed by making natural processes work more effectively and operate as if they are younger.

Collagen and elastin are two critical proteins within the skin responsible for their bounce, firmness, and wrinkles. With the aid of red-light therapy, the production of these two essential proteins can be increased, and the skin can become firmer with fewer wrinkles.

Red-light Therapy Benefits:

- Minimizes the lines and wrinkles
- Shrink pore size
- Improves the skin tone and texture

- Reduces Black Spots

- Repairs sun-damaged skin

- Reduces redness

- Stimulates collagen production

Aging is unavoidable; but, you can do something about it with devices like red-light therapy and promote skiing Red-light therapy follows more than 40 years of research and has made countless men and women without invasive procedures look younger.

It is a treatment that can stay in your skin and make a difference.

Red-light Therapy for Anti-Aging

Red-light therapy is a form of LED light therapy, also called photorejuvenation, for anti-aging purposes. Light-emitting dioceses applied to the skin are used to encourage younger, healthier skin. Red-light therapy is entirely natural and triggers a body reaction to improve your skin from within.

NASA has researched and developed this skin treatment and was initially used to test the plant reaction under LEDs. The mechanism revealed it was growing more rapidly and eventually verified its efficacy in human cells. While plants and human cells are different, light has naturally improved skin conditions at the ideal wavelength.

Yes, the red dye is used for recovery and several other problems, such as pain management (back pain, tendonitis, tennis elbow, etc.). When in conjunction with infrared lights, the cycle is even more effective because infrared penetrates deeper.

As regards skincare, your skin absorbs light, stimulating elastin and collagen production. Such two proteins are naturally extremely important for the strength and elasticity of your skin.

The production of elastin and collagen decreases as we age, plus the small veins that bring nutrients into the skin surface are even smaller. Red light renews cells and makes these veins bring more blood, more nutrients into your skin.

Red-light therapy has a cumulative effect. The softer and smoother the skin is, the more you use it. Generally, treatments take about 15 to 30 minutes for the entire face, but of course, it is possible to focus your efforts on some areas of your face: crow feet, lip corners, neck, etc.

Wrinkles and fine lines are packed with collagen again, and you'll be pleased to obtain this great tone and luster on your back.

One type of LED light therapy uses blue light to combat acne. Hyperpigmentation is the green light.

The beauty of it is that it is not surgery, and after all, you do not need a lot of creams and lotions. Although only available from skin clinics, dermatologists, and spas in the first place, red-light therapy equipment is now on the public market.

The costs of such devices vary ($100-$ 400) but are worthwhile given the savings in other care products and much more affordable than professional office sessions.

Keeping significant skin is about producing collagen, and this can be achieved in many ways: Vitamins A, E, C, and several acids and peel therapies and IPL fantastic collagen stimulation.

Most of these treatments rely upon inflammation to increase the skin cell turnover and thereby plump the skin. Still, a new fantastic treatment is available under the Stimulating Collagen banner, which does not harm the skin in any way.

Although light therapy has been around for some time, it is considered the latest advance in skin treatment technology. Red-light therapy can fight the signs of aging, including wrinkles and dry skin.

It's just like plant photosynthesis. Just as crops use chlorophyll to transform sunlight into cellular building blocks, Red-light activates natural intracellular chemical processes that generate cellular turns and collagen and elastin fiber development.

Red light activates skin ATP output in the mitochondria; the mitochondria release cell production energy.

This release of energy increases the output of healthy cells that replace the damaged cells. Unlike other light therapies such as IPL and Laser, this procedure does not depend on heat but instead receives an energy boost for the cells. It is essential to understand that this treatment does not contain UV rays, so it is 100% safe, with no known contra-indications.

As mentioned previously, light therapy in medical settings has been used to improve wound healing for many years, and beauty salons and spas have been introduced as the price of the equipment has fallen.

The anti-aging light spectrum is 615 nm and 640 nm, which contains RED light. The receptors in the brain are activated by light at specific wavelengths; different frequencies cause different responses. Red light has been demonstrated to encourage the production and counteract the effects of aging and sun damage by collagen and elastin in the skin.

In conjunction with the University of Pavia, clinical tests reported 20.2% less wrinkle frequency, 24.7% better skin moisturization, and 15.1% better skin smoothness. The process uses wavelengths in the visible light range to transmit light into the layers of the skin. This light energy activates a cellular activity reaction called photo modulation when applied to the skin.

The light is absorbed by the cell and dispersed evenly to stimulate the cellular collagen that produces skin rejuvenation and skin healing mechanisms. Ideally, these procedures would be done at least 4–5 days a week for 4-6 weeks, and you will begin to see a change in skin tone and texture by the end of this treatment period.

The key to successful red-light treatment is to know that time is needed. Bear in mind that not only do you turn the clock back, but you also slow down the aging process.

RED lighting machines initially targeted the face, but the red light is now available to treat the whole body in the form of collagen beds. It's a fascinating development as often we spend a lot of time and money on the skin, but the rest of the body is missing. At the age of 50, you can find that the skin starts to sag throughout the entire body.

Collagen beds help slow down this aging process. The' next big thing after Botox ' is being promoted. There are numerous other advantages and anti-aging. A headache can be alleviated, and poor circulation can be improved since Red-light relaxes the blood vessels to allow more vital blood flow.

Light is also treated for depression and seasonal imbalance (SAD). The use of light therapy also supports soft tissue injuries and sprains. New benefits are regularly discovered, including reducing symptoms of sexual dysfunction, although these statements may not be scientifically validated.

Red-light Therapy Encourages Collagen and Elastin Production

The unique structure of your skin consists of two key proteins: collagen and elastin. Those two essential components in the layers of your skin ensure solid and healthy skin integrity. When they age, your collagen and elastin can be affected as production slows down and is damaged and broken by exposure to free radicals and the oxidation process.

To maintain healthy and youthful skin, you need to keep vital collagen, elastin, and healthy production. When production increases and you build up a large amount of these two essential proteins, your taint will react better and safer. Increased production of collagen can help reduce wrinkles and make the skin look younger.

NASA invented Red-light Therapy, also called LED Light Therapy, to significantly speed up the space healing process. More work has shown that LED red-light therapy enhances collagen and synthesis of elastin and improves cellular gain.

Red LED lights of 625 to 660 nanometers are easily absorbed into the skin and penetrate deep into your skin's layers. These beneficial longitudes energize your cells, repair the damage, speed up healing, renew, regenerate, and increase collagen and elastin production.

Red LED light treatment is a gentle option for skin rejuvenation and reduction of body pain. Research shows that this technique helps your skin tremendously and fills your cells with repair properties.

Falts have been shown to decrease skin tone, age and scar, skin firmness, pores reduction, and defects reduction. This advanced technology is used in spas, physicians, clinics and is also available at home. Some systems have been withdrawn from the FDA as medical devices and are eligible for home use.

It is an increasingly popular technology because of its ease and efficiency. Find devices that expose the nanometer range of the wavelength to ensure successful results. You must be vigilant because specific devices do not reveal their nanometers and use wavelengths that benefit the skin.

You can expect dramatic improvements in the appearance of your skin by using a high-quality system. Improving your production of collagen and elastin helps your skin look best and keeps it youthful.

People worldwide use the healing and repairing abilities of light to improve skin health and appearance. Something as basic as light provides tremendous skin refreshments and regenerative properties that shock even those most dismissive of skeptics, including dermatologists, hospitals, and universities.

Specific wavelengths can penetrate deep into the skin and tissue and are readily accepted by the body with their power to heal. These exact wavelengths of LED (light-emitting diode) ignite more than 24 positive cellular response levels.

They stimulate mitochondria, cell energy, and cell metabolism, which generate new, healthy collagen. As the energy within the cell increases, it can work optimally to produce a more beautiful taint.

Wavelengths are measured in nanometers (nm) that create a plethora of beautiful colors. Each of these colors is important when it comes to skin healing. The red LEDs are very beneficial for cellular skins, encouraging treatment, repair, regeneration, rejuvenation, and relaxation, from 610 to 660 nm to-infrared LEDs at 880 nm (naked to the human eye).

Collagen is the most abundant protein in the body and a vital component in the skin. Collagen binds the cells together, creating a complex fiber network to bounce the skin and make it more elastic. LED light therapy has the rare ability to enhance collagen production.

Hair with damaged or brittle collagen fibers looks older and shows lines, wrinkles, rough texture, and a lack of firmness. When people age, the body produces less collagen and holds collagen fibers healthier.

LED light therapy improves skin health, making it look smoother, more robust, and healthier by increasing the synthesis and repairing damaged fibers. It is as easy as exposing the skin to red-light therapy and stimulation near. Restoring wavelengths penetrate the skin, permeate and induce various positive responses.

Red-light therapy is a natural, non-invasive and safe option for improving skin appearance and behavior. Although an effective anti-aging instrument, this therapy takes time to see dramatic results.

Chapter 3: How is Red-light Therapy Used?

How is a red-light treatment utilized?

As far back as the underlying trials in space, several clinical investigations and much research have been directed to decide whether RLT has health advantages.

Numerous investigations have had promising outcomes, yet the advantages of red-light treatment are as yet a wellspring of discussion. The Centers for Medicare and Medicaid Services (CMS), for instance, has confirmed that there isn't sufficient proof to show that these gadgets are superior to at present existing medications for treating wounds, ulcers, and agony.

Extra clinical research is expected to demonstrate that RLT is compelling. Right now, nonetheless, there's some proof to propose that RLT may have the accompanying advantages:

- advances wound mending and tissue fix
- improves hair development in individuals with androgenic alopecia
- help for the transient treatment of carpal passage disorder
- animates mending of moderate recuperating wounds, similar to diabetic foot ulcers
- diminishes psoriasis injuries
- helps with temporary alleviation of torment and morning solidness in individuals with rheumatoid joint pain

- lessens a portion of the symptoms of disease medicines, including oral mucositisTrusted Source

- improves skin composition and constructs collagenTrusted Source to reduce wrinkles

- repairs sun

- keeps repeating mouth blisters from herpes simplex infection diseases

- improves the soundness of joints in individuals with degenerative osteoarthritis of the knee

- decreases scars

- mitigates torment and inflammationTrusted Source in individuals with suffering in the Achilles ligaments

RLT isn't supported or secured by insurance agencies for these conditions because of the absence of adequate proof. A couple of insurance agencies presently spread the utilization of RLT to counteract oral mucositis during malignant growth treatment.

Be that as it may, does red-light treatment truly work?

While the web is frequently buzzing with news about marvel medications for pretty much every wellbeing condition, red-light treatment indeed isn't a fix just for everything. RLT is viewed as a trial for most situations.

There are constrained to-no proof indicating that red-light treatment does the accompanying:

- treats sadness, regular full of feeling issues, and post-birth anxiety
- initiates the lymphatic framework to help "detoxify" the body
- supports the invulnerable framework
- lessens cellulite
- helps in weight reduction
- treats back or neck torment
- battles periodontitis and dental contaminations
- fixes skin inflammation
- treats malignancy

Note that when RLT is utilized with malignancy medicines, the light is just used to initiate another prescription. Other light treatments have been used to help with a portion of the conditions above. For example, thinks about have discovered that white light treatment is more successful at treating side effects of misery than red light. Blue light treatment is all the more generally utilized for skin inflammation, with constrained viability.

Are there comparable treatment alternatives?

Red-light wavelengths aren't the primary wavelengths to be read for therapeutic purposes. Blue light, green light, and a blend of various wavelengths have additionally been the subject of comparative trials in people.

There are different sorts of light-based treatments accessible. You can get some information about:

- laser medications
- regular daylight
- blue or green light treatment
- sauna light treatment
- bright light B (UVB)
- psoralen and bright light A (PUVA)

Picking a supplier

Many tanning salons, rec centers, and nearby day spas offer RLT for corrective applications. You can likewise discover FDA-endorsed gadgets online that you can buy and use at home. Costs will change. You can have a go at utilizing these gadgets to battle the indications of maturing, similar to age spots, scarcely discernible differences, and wrinkles. However, make a point to peruse the directions cautiously. Look at specific gadgets on the web.

For more focus on RLT, you'll have to see a dermatologist first. You may require a few medicines before you notice any distinction.

To treat genuine ailments similar to malignancy, joint pain, and psoriasis, you should make a meeting with your primary care physician to talk about your alternatives.

Symptoms

Red-light treatment is viewed as protected and accessible. Nonetheless, there have been reports of consumption and rankling from utilizing RLT units. A couple of individuals created consumption in the wake of nodding off with the unit set up, while others encountered consumption because of broken wires or gadget erosion.

There's additionally a potential danger of harm to the eyes. Although more secure on the eyes than conventional lasers, appropriate eye assurance should consistently be utilized while experiencing red-light treatment.

Takeaway

RLT has indicated promising outcomes in treating some skin conditions. However, inside established researchers, there's very little agreement about the treatment's advantages. In light of the momentum inquire, you may find that RLT is a decent device to add to your healthy skin routine. Continuously check with your PCP or dermatologist before taking a stab at something new.

You can, without much of a stretch, buy red-light gadgets on the web; however, it's ideal to hear a specialist's point of view on any indications before you attempt to self-treat. Remember that RLT isn't FDA-endorsed for most conditions or secured by insurance agencies. Any actual situation, similar to psoriasis, joint inflammation, slow-mending wounds, or agony, ought to be looked at by a specialist.

There is some proof to back up many of these cases; however, RLT is no supernatural occurrence fix.

Anybody considering the treatment ought to likewise find a way to advance skin wellbeing. Inappropriate utilization of RLT may again cause some reactions.

Any individual who is unsure whether RLT is directly for them should converse with their primary care physician.

How it functions

RLT is a precise technique, including presenting the body to low wavelength red light. Low-level laser light treatment is another name for the procedure; however, RLT might be increasingly regular.

This red light is normal and can infiltrate profound into the skin, where the cells can ingest and utilize it.

As an investigation in the diary Seminars in Cutaneous Medicine and SurgeryTrusted Source notes, mitochondria in the skin cells can ingest these light particles. It can enable the cells to deliver more adenosine triphosphate, which is the vitality hotspot for all cells.

Numerous specialists property the potential positive advantages of RLT to this capacity. With this additional vitality, the cells might have the option to react better to harm and revive themselves.

Although early research encompasses RLT, there is still no decisive proof that it is a valuable treatment. Numerous investigations show that the therapy has guaranteed, yet progressively broad clinical examinations in people will help decide the potential uses of RLT.

There are a few potential advantages of RLT, which we will cover in the segments beneath.

Hair development

A little report in the Journal of Cosmetic and Laser Therapy investigated the impact of low-level light on individuals with alopecia.

The examination uncovered that individuals who got RLT had improved hair thickness, contrasted with those in a control group.

The creators note that the impact was gainful when individuals applied light in wavelengths of both 665 nanometres (nm) and 808 nm.

Be that as it may, this was a little report, and progressively broad clinical investigations will help offer sponsorship to these cases.

Decreasing torment

RLT may likewise be a viable treatment for torment in individuals with specific conditions.

The European Journal of Physical and Rehabilitation Medicine has paid attention to several aftereffects encompassing RLT use. One of these was musculoskeletal issues.

The exploration showed that RLT could adequately lessen torment in grown-ups with the various musculoskeletal issue. The analysts note that professionals who adhere to the particular dose suggestions appear to build the adequacy of the treatment.

Improving bone recuperation

A survey in the Journal of Photochemistry and PhotobiologyTrusted Source analyzes the potential for RLT in treating facial bone imperfections.

The specialists' outcomes demonstrate that RLT may help quicken recuperating after treatment for facial bone deformities. The audit additionally takes note that the treatment decreased irritation and agony during the procedure.

Be that as it may, the analysts called for an increasingly standardized way to decide if the treatment was successful.

Mitigating benefits

As research in the diary AIMS BiophysicsTrusted Source notes, many of the conditions that RLT treats have their foundations in aggravation.

Although the careful explanation isn't yet clear, RLT has huge calming impacts on the body. These impacts are both neighborhoods, where experts apply the light, and foundational, in different tissues and organs in the body.

The scientists clarify that the accommodating calming impacts of RLT, and the potential uses for this treatment, are rich.

Further research may assist us with comprehension on the off chance that it might help with interminable fiery issues, for example,

Alzheimer's ailment

- heftiness
- type 2 diabetes
- alopecia areata
- immune system thyroiditis, or irritation of the thyroid
- psoriasis
- joint inflammation
- tendinitis, or irritation of the ligaments

Once more, the examination is as yet primer. Be that as it may, the mitigating impact of RLT is promising.

Past examinations have focused on the significance of the particular wavelengths that individuals use to focus on their skin.

Nonetheless, as the audit in Seminars in Cutaneous Medicine and SurgeryTrusted Source clarifies, the gathered research found that much of the time, quite specific wavelengths had moderately little effect during treatment.

The recurrence for most RLT sessions will commonly differ inside a range, like the wavelengths in the Journal of Photochemistry and PhotobiologyTrusted Source paper.

Potential reactions

RLT is a standard procedure. It opens the skin to levels of light that are not hurtful — dissimilar to UV light originating from the sun.

Along these lines, there is no danger of symptoms from experiencing RLT. Be that as it may, an expert with little experience or somebody who opens themselves to a lot of the treatment may cause tissue and cell harm.

Items for use at home may likewise prompt abuse, making harm the skin, consumption, or harm to unprotected eyes.

Expenses and protection inclusion

RLT is accessible in various exercise centers, day spas, and tanning salons.

RLT has a generally low working expense. It is likewise not a prescription in the conventional sense, so it is broadly accessible. Numerous foundations may offer RLT rooms or lights, including:

- exercise centers

- day spas

- tanning salons

- wellbeing focuses

- saunas

- dermatology workplaces

Numerous organizations additionally offer items that utilization focused on red-light lights as a spot mending device. Anybody obtaining such gadgets for use at home should check to ensure that the gadget conveys red-light inside the powerful wavelengths before finishing the buy.

There is no protection inclusion for the general act of RLT. In any case, a few dermatologists may offer focused on RLT applications. Any individual concerned about a skin issue that RLT may help should see their primary care physician for a referral.

Red-light treatment (RLT) is a treatment that may help skin, muscle tissue, and different pieces of your body mend. It opens you to low degrees of red or closes infrared light. Infrared light is a sort of vitality your eyes can't see, yet your body can feel as warmth. Red-light is like infrared, yet you can see it.

Red-light treatment is likewise called low-level laser treatment (LLLT), low-control laser treatment (LPLT), and photobiomodulation (PBM).

How Does Red-light Therapy Work?

With red-light treatment, you open your skin to light, gadget, or laser with a red light. A piece of your phone called mitochondria, at times called the "control generators" of your phones, absorb it and make more vitality. A few specialists think this assists cells with fixing themselves and become more advantageous—this spikes recuperating in skin and muscle tissue.

Things You're Not Telling Your Doctor

Indeed, even the most wellbeing-conscious among us may not tell our PCPs every bit of relevant information when we see them.

Simplicity Secondary Progressive MS With Lifestyle Changes

Medication isn't the best way to treat optional dynamic different sclerosis (SPMS). Diet, workout, and additional changes to your day-by-day schedule could likewise help decrease your side effects.

Chapter 4: But Does Red-light Therapy Really Work?

Does RLT Work: The Scientific Proof/Benefits

To answer the question, RLT works. As scientific research has shown and proven, using it has various benefits, many of which we shall discuss at length in this chapter.

RLT works by shining a brilliant and therapeutic red light on the skin, stimulating ATP molecules production. This metabolic process helps cellular healing and rejuvenation.

Scores of research studies have shown that when used safely and consistently, the resulting biochemical process caused by exposure to red-light therapy has the following potential benefits:

RLT Benefits the Skin

Various studies have concluded that controlled use of safe red-light is immensely beneficial for the skin.

RLT therapy enhances the overall health of the skin. As we discussed earlier, when the red-light impacts skin cells (where it stimulates the production of ATP), this enhanced production leads to overall cellular well-being, which effectively translates to smoother, acne-free, healthier skin, boosting collagen production means wrinkle-free skin. Because of enhanced cell health, better healing abilities, and less skin scaring.

Many professionals, dermatologists, celebrities, estheticians, and influential publications such as Elle, CNN, and others have publicly noted the positive effects red-light therapy has on the skin.

Here is how the process works to enhance your skin's enhanced well-being to enhance your understanding of how red-light therapy leads to your skin's enhanced well-being.

How this works

Shining a controlled wavelength of red light is the essence of red-light therapy. The red-light treatment, exposing your skin to these wavelengths(660-850 nm) of light, is safe because even without shining a red light on the cells, they can absorb from the environment these wavelengths of light and use it to power cellular functionality.

By this process, your cells receive the wavelength of pure red light to stimulate ATP production, leading to better skin functionality (remember that the skin is an organ, too, in fact, one of the largest and most important organs).

When the skin cells function better, and when the cells can circulate well within the various skin layers and the Electron Transport Chain, it leads to lower oxidation. Lower oxidation means an efficient cellular energy production process, better circulation, functionality, reduced skin inflammation, better protection from harmful rays, and improved skin appearance and health.

Regarding increasing cells circulation within the various skin layers, a *research study conducted by Maria Emília de Abreu Chaves et al.* noted that continued controlled use of red-light therapy in any form—even a handheld device used at home—increases circulation by ensuring that the cells function effectively. The tissues receive the energy, nutritional, and oxygen support they need to function optimally.

Moreover, because the process also reduces oxidative stress on the cells, it enhances the skin's ability to detoxify itself—a lesser need for 'skin detoxes' and products—and heal wounds and scar tissues better and much faster.

RLT is beneficial for the skin in many, many ways.

For instance:

The anti-inflammatory aspect: When you shine a therapeutic grade red light on your skin, it stimulates a biochemical process that enhances your skin cells' ability to create energy for themselves, the overall skin layer, and for other parts of the body. Because all our organs are interconnected, when the cells on the skin heal and rejuvenate themselves better and faster, thereby bringing about a healing effect, this effect passes on to other areas and parts of the body.

One aspect of the healing effect red-light therapy has on the skin cells is that it significantly reduces inflammation and stress. Again, when you shine a therapeutic grade red light on skin cells, it enhances their functionality. It means that the cells receive better energy, blood, and oxygen flow, which means an enhanced ability to heal, repair, and rejuvenate.

To be specific, a research study conducted by Dr. Michael Hamblin noted, "skin cells consider the wavelengths used for red-light and near infrared-light therapy a form of mild stress. When you expose these skin cells to this form of mild stress, it activates their need to self-protect (and protect you too). When the cells are in the self-protect mode, they function more efficiently and are very adept at creating the antioxidants they need to fight any inflammatory effect caused by the mild stress."

When it comes to reducing inflammation, red-light therapy is so effective that *one study published in Medical Science* noted that RLT treatment has a very therapeutic effect on post-surgery inflammation. Reduced post-surgery inflammation leads to better pain relief. Minor wound swelling and irritation, quicker healing, and recovery times, which means with consultation, red-light therapy after surgery can be beneficial for wound management, stimulating the cells to work better and heal quicker.

A *research study conducted by Lee JH, et al.* concluded that using red-light therapy on the mouth — exposing the periodontal cells to treatment — leads to decrease inflammation and enhanced cells ability to stave off toxins such as P. gingivalis and E. coli (prevalent mouth toxins).

We cannot talk about inflammation—and the effect red-light therapy has on its reduction and leave out mentioning its effect on musculoskeletal soreness or muscle soreness.

A *research study published in 2008* noted that controlled heliotherapy—as a reminder, RLT is a form of heliotherapy, the controlled use of light for healing purposes—significantly reduces symptoms of muscle soreness. In *another research study from Brazil*, researchers concluded that using a red-light therapy machine before a workout led to a significant decrease in post-workout pain and muscle soreness/inflammation.

RLT Enhances Sleep

Better sleep means better rest and, therefore, more energy and increased productivity in your day. Red-light therapy has proven effective in improving your sleep patterns, enhancing your circadian rhythms, normalizing cells' ability to produce melatonin. This hormone whose primary production is to help the body control your sleep-and-wake upcycle).

Morita T., Tokura H conducted a research study to determine the effect Red-light therapy sessions during the day may have on the body's ability to produce melatonin. She decided that exposure to pure red light during the day led to enhanced melatonin production and a rationalized circadian rhythm. This congruency can only mean one thing: red-light therapy sessions during the day will lead to better sleep and rest.

To enhance your understanding of how red-light therapy improves sleep, here is how the process works.

How this works

Let's start by agreeing on one thing: poor sleep patterns have negative short and long-term consequences and effects.

For example:

Poor sleep patterns affect hormonal balance, which then affects our mood/wellbeing. Poor sleep patterns also lead to low energy, which means decreased output and productivity, which by itself brings a ton of negative consequences such as an inability to achieve your aims.

Additionally, the sense of 'chronic tiredness' can lead to mental health complications such as anxiety, stress, depression, and attendant conditions such as rapid weight gain or loss. It has also increased the risk of type 2 diabetes and insulin imbalances that disrupt your body's ability to determine when it needs sustenance.

Some research studies have concluded that poor sleep can decrease cognitive function, such as a low attention span and decreased mental clarity.

Outlining how abnormal sleep patterns decrease the overall percentage of your wellbeing was important because it created a background that will help you understand how red-light therapy ensures better sleep.

The first thing you should note is that our sleep cycles are light-dependent. It means that when it comes to sleeping, i.e., when it comes to how your body decides when it needs rest in the form of sleep, light is the determinant factor. The body uses natural (and artificial) light to determine when to produce the hormones it needs to ensure that it [as a machine] has an operationally effective circadian system/rhythm.

Modern lives are full of artificial lights, think bulbs, and screens. These conditions can lead to a confused circadian pattern, one that throws your sleep cycle off balance, thereby making it harder for you to fall asleep naturally, rest well, and wake up feeling refreshed and rejuvenated.

Secondly, it's important to point out the negative effect some lights have on our circadian rhythm and ability to sleep and rest; for specificity, we shall concentrate on blue light.

Exposure to blue light is widespread in our daily lives on screens such as televisions, monitors, laptops, tablets, phones, etc. Since most of us have grown accustomed to blue light exposure in the evening and long into the night, our bodies have learned to interpret this to mean it should remain awake because it's light outside.

Various clinical research studies have demonstrated and concluded that having red-light therapy sessions in the evening has the potential to improve your sleep patterns. The science behind this is as logical as logic is! Pure red light has a lower temperature; exposing your body to such wavelengths in the evening communicates that the light has changed and that it should prepare for rest by producing the necessary hormone, melatonin.

In 2013, Taiwanese researchers sought to determine the state of brain activity (electroencephalography EEG) before, during, and after red-light therapy sessions. They did this by analyzing the EEGs of study participants. This research study concluded that exposure to a therapeutic, pure red light in the evening effectively combat common sleep disorders.

In another *research study published in 2014*, researchers noted that patients suffering from traumatic brain injury (TBI) experienced minor PTSD after red-light therapy, reported better sleep patterns, and improved brain function.

In another Brazilian research study published in 2018, researchers concluded that red-light therapy proved highly effective against sleep disorders and other no-sleep-related complications such as migraines.

As mentioned earlier, part of its effectiveness as a form of "alternative sleep therapy" is its effect on the signals that trigger melatonin production. Because pure grade red and near-infrared lights have a low temperature, exposure to them at ideal times of the day can positively affect natural melatonin production.

The logical conclusion from the various research studies mentioned is that red-light therapy is an alternative sleep therapy. Lying in pure red light in the evening can make it easier to fall asleep and sleep better.

The specific relation called "How red-light therapy leads to improved sleep" *research by Margaret N., Michael H.* has shown the following results: after 18, 1-hour, daily red-light therapy sessions, patients suffering from traumatic brain injury slept for an hour longer and woke up feeling more rested and refreshed.

RLT has Weight Loss Benefits

First off, when it comes to weight loss, nothing beats good-ol' healthy eating and consistent engagement in some form of physical activity such as exercise. With that noted, we can do various ways to enhance weight and fat loss. Some examples include practicing intermittent fasting—eating within a specific hour window—taking weight loss supplements such as garcinia cambogia, and detoxing. RLT can also be effective as an alternative weight loss strategy you can couple with healthy eating and adequate exercise and enhance your body's ability to burn fat.

Various research studies have shown red-light therapy's positive influence on weight loss, gain, or retainment. In particular, researchers have noted that red-light therapy is a practical, alternative weight loss strategy because its effects act upon the adipocytes cells, the cells in your body responsible for storing fat.

In 2011, Paolillo FR, Borghi-Silva A, et al. published a study detailing what the researchers discovered after subjecting study participants—women aged 25-55—to treadmill exercises and red-light therapy. The study revolved around categorizing the participants into two categories: those who engaged in treadmill running and those that did treadmill running and two sessions of red-light therapy each week, with the study measure being to determine how red-light therapy influences cellulite.

These researchers demonstrated dramatic differences between the two study groups. The starkest of these differences was that the group engaged in treadmill/cardio exercises and two red-light therapy each week showed dramatic improvement of thigh cellulite. The researchers then concluded that engaging in exercise and RLT leads to an aesthetically pleasing body and increased fat loss.

In 2012, the *International Journal of Endocrinology*—the study of medicine concerning hormones and glands—published a research study where researchers concluded that light influences our eating patterns and that this can itself influence our hunger and satiety levels.

These researchers concluded that when your hunger and satiety hormones and signals are out of whack', the effect is a decreased ability to regulate when [and when not] you eat. This reduced ability can lead to the development of conditions such as binge eating and various hormone-regulations conditions such as type 2 diabetes and a cellular attachment to storing fat in the form of lipids. Red-light and near infrared-light therapy increases cellular activity, which effectively means that as cells work better, their ability to release fat lipids increases. When this happens, i.e., when the cells release fat lipids, the effect is weight/fat loss. Coupled with healthy eating and exercise, red-light therapy can intensely improve your weight loss journey.

To enhance your understanding of how red-light therapy improves weight loss, here is how the process works.

How this works

Let's recap what you now understand about red-light therapy. You know that this alternative therapy works by delivering pure red light on the skin, which causes increased cellular activity. You also know that once red light stimulates increased production of ATP, it ensures your cells operate optimally and as effectively as possible.

Red-light therapy works so effectively as an alternative form of weight loss therapy because it activates enhanced activity in adipocytes, the body's fat regulating cells. When red and near-infrared lights contact the skin, the resultant biochemical reaction triggers increased activity in these fat cells that, when activated, cause the cells to release any excess fat (lipids) they may be carrying unnecessarily.

In addition to this, researchers have concluded that the effectiveness of RLT as an alternative weight-loss management system comes from its ability to regulate the production of various hunger hormones [but specifically ghrelin and leptin].

Tons of research findings fully support red-light therapy as an alternative weight loss strategy/system that, coupled with healthy eating and adequate exercise, can significantly lose fat and increase metabolism.

One part of wanting to lose weight is sculpting the 'body of your dreams.' To this end, you may use various therapies at your disposal, such as multiple body sculpting techniques and, in some cases, targeted surgeries.

There is scientific evidence proving that using RLT with weight loss and other good-health strategies can significantly improve your chances of losing fat and help get the body you have always wanted.

Handheld RLT devices are an incredibly effective way to 'contour' the body simply because they allow for better targeting and maneuverability. By allowing for better targeting of specific 'fatty' areas such as love handles, thighs, and underarms. Using pure red light to influence increased activity in areas that tend to carry fat, your body releases the lipids within cells, making the weight loss process more manageable.

In *one study conducted in 2011 and results published in the Journal of Obesity Surgery*, researchers concluded that red-light therapy could lead to a slimmer waistline after a double-blind study. The study involved allowing participants access to 635-80nm red-light therapy sessions for four weeks. The researchers focused on the effect these therapy sessions had on the circumference of the waistline. Their study concluded that exposure to red light at the wavelengths above has excellent potential as a waistline sculpting tool.

Various other studies support the findings of the study as mentioned above. One such study appears in *Lasers in Surgery Medicine*. In this research study, researchers sought to know the effectiveness of RLT as a targeted weight loss tool—how effective it is at helping one lose weight in targeted areas. After offering participants red-light and near infrared-light therapy sessions, the researchers found that these led to significant body fat loss in critical areas such as the thighs, underarms, etc.

In another study published in 2013, researchers determined that exposure to pure red-light at 635nm led to contoured thighs and hips. Some participants in this study saw a reduction of up to 2.99 inches of their augmented body size.

Chapter 5: For Which Kind of Treatment is Indicate RTL?

Red-light therapy is a unique yet straightforward option that employs red-light to treat various health disorders. Red and near-infrared light have low wavelengths to penetrate deep into the skin, allowing the cells to use and leverage their power.

Through the profound penetration effect, RLT bypasses the harmful step of multiple other therapies involving damage caused to the superficial layers of skin. The light from RLT devices penetrates about 5 mm beneath the surface of the skin. Let us explain how red-light therapy works.

Natural light is essential for all living beings, including human beings, to survive on our planet. Air, food, and light are the most vital components of life on earth. The human body is a powerful natural machine made up of billions of cells performing a vast range of complex functions. Each of these billions of cells needs energy to function normally.

Energy is produced in our cells continuously through the process of cellular respiration. Red and near-infrared light play a crucial role in this process of energy production at the cellular level. So, how does red light help in cellular respiration?

The answer lies in one of the essential cellular structures called mitochondria, commonly referred to as the "powerhouses of cells." Mitochondria are unique cellular structures that affect everything we do, although they are not visible to the naked eye. Mitochondria form a crucial component in adenosine triphosphate (ATP) production. It is referred to as the "energy currency of life." The number of mitochondria in each cell varies between 1-2 and multiple thousands, depending on the function of each cell.

So, what is ATP? ATPs are energy-carrying molecules found in all living cells. The amount of ATP produced and used by each cell type depends on the function and needs of each cell. For example, muscle cells need a lot more ATPs than other cells in the body as they are used intensively for doing all kinds of physical work.

ATP is created through cellular respiration, a highly efficient and complex natural metabolic process that involves naturally-available ingredients like oxygen, light, water, and food. Mitochondria is an essential component of the ATP production process. Red-light wavelengths stimulate mitochondrial functioning resulting in increased and efficient energy production processes within each body cell.

Studies have shown that mitochondria can absorb red and near-infrared light particles, which helps the cells produce more ATP than before. Effectively, RLT produces a biochemical effect in cells so that the functioning of mitochondria is strengthened, resulting in cells being able to produce more ATP. Consequently, more energy is available for the body.

The photons in red (and near-infrared) light excite electrons leading to the break-up of nitric oxide bonds. Consequently, the protons are available more freely to combine with oxygen for increased production of ATP. Your body feels rejuvenated with increased production of ATP through cellular production.

Therefore, red and near-infrared light stimulates mitochondria and breaks up nitric oxide bonds resulting in increased ATP production and reduced oxidative stress. In addition to facilitating the increased production of ATP for increased energy availability to perform better, the other important principles of red-light therapy are:

They reduced oxidative stress through improved production of antioxidants. Natural red-light and near-infrared-light are known to promote the production of antioxidants. Help reduce oxidative stress (if left unresolved, this condition can lead to premature cell death), cause muscle fatigue, cell injury, inflammation, and joint pain. Antioxidants also play an essential role in producing special enzymes called heat proteins that help protect cells from oxidative stress.

Improved blood circulation - Multiple studies have also demonstrated that RLT helps increase blood circulation, which means tissues receive more oxygen and nutrients, leading to enhanced performance and better healing.

Some of the proven benefits of RLT include:

- Reduced inflammation and joint pain

- Increased collagen production

- Improved sleep

- Weight loss facilitation

- Improved muscle recovery and physical performance

Other names including: also know RLT

- Low-level light therapy (LLLT)

- Photobiomodulation (PBM)

- Cold laser therapy

- Soft laser therapy

- Biostimulation

- Low-power laser therapy (LPLT)

- Photonic stimulation

In some cases, RLT is used as an activating agent in photosensitizing medications; it is called photodynamic therapy. Red-light therapy has found multiple applications in the medical and cosmetic fields. In salons, RLT is used for cosmetic purposes such as skin tightening, skin lightening, etc.

In medicine, RLT is employed as an effective supplementary (and sometimes, even as a primary) therapy to treat severe disorders like psoriasis, chronic and slow-healing wounds and reduce the side effects of chemotherapy.

While numerous studies have demonstrated the efficacy of RLT to treat various medical conditions, a lot more research is going on in this field, driven by promising results observed in current studies. Yet, a lot more work needs to be done before we can completely understand and harness the power of RTL optimally.

Red-light Therapy for Fat Loss and Weight Management

Losing pounds and inches is one of the most sought-after elements of modern-day life, thanks to an explosion in social media of both celebrities and ordinary people undergoing makeovers.

An increasing number of people are being motivated to shed excess weight and achieve weight loss goals. However, it is easier said than done. Exercising and dieting are challenging for most people and don't work effectively for some of us. A bit of help from any quarter is always welcome when it comes to weight loss. Red-light therapy seems to provide this much-needed relief.

Red-light therapy has revolutionized the ideas behind fat and weight loss. Until the discovery of RLT, it was believed that it was impossible to choose a particular body part from which we want to lose fat or weight. For example, you can run a marathon. However, there is no guarantee that only your legs and thighs will lose fat. Similarly, you can do multiple stomach crunches. But there is no way of confirming that only your stomach area will lose fat or weight.

Now, thanks to some revolutionary findings based on RLT research, experts opine that targeted fat loss is possible. So, how does RLT facilitate fat and weight loss? RLT reduces oxidative stress and stimulates increased production of ATP for more energy. Research has also shown that RLT affects fat cells, which are biologically termed adipocytes. RLT affects adipocytes in such a way as to disperse lipids. Experts opine that RLT helps the body wash away or drain away fat cells, resulting in fat and/or weight loss.

Here is what experts believe happens with RLT that facilitates weight loss. Red-light therapy penetrates about 5 mm beneath the skin's surface, bypassing the susceptible epidermal layer. Red light directly targets the skin layers well below the epidermis, stimulating the mitochondria in these cells for increased ATP, and consequently, energy production. Further, the near-infrared light is absorbed by skin tissues, which results in the break up of water molecules, resulting in the release of toxins and fats.

Here are some other ways that RLT helps in fat and weight loss:

Reduces hunger levels - Reducing hunger is one of the most effective ways to deal with excessive food intake, directly affecting weight management. Before the advent of RLT, we could only reduce hunger by undergoing the hazardous procedure of gastric bypass surgery or bariatric surgery. Recent studies demonstrate that RLT can help reduce hunger pangs and the urge to eat.

Studies showed that RLT shows promise in controlling and managing hunger hormones in the human body, namely ghrelin and leptin. Leptin helps to decrease appetite, and ghrelin works in the opposite direction by increasing thirst and hunger. Controlling these two hormones can help you manage your eating habits to prevent weight and fat gain. RLT is believed to be a safe and non-invasive approach to reduce hunger pangs to control weight. RLT is especially useful to maintain body weight after you have lost a couple of pounds.

Reduced Cellulite - RLT, which combines red and near-infrared light, has proven to help in weight loss by lowering cellulite-producing fat pockets in the body. Cellulite is formed through the build-up of unhealthy elastin, collagen, and excess fat in the layers of the skin.

RLT replenishes and rejuvenates collagen production by enhancing the growth of fibroblasts, which are responsible for collagen production and help tighten the skin by increasing collagen movement through the walls of cells. Therefore, RLT helps reduce cellulite and helps to tighten the skin, ensuring you get the best weight-loss look.

RLT combats cellulite in another way too. One of the primary contributing factors of cellulite development is compromised blood circulation that results in reduced diffusion of essential nutrients to the affected parts, which causes a weakening of the skin's connective tissues. RLT has demonstrated that it can improve blood circulation and promote the health of the blood vessels in the areas where cellulite develops.

RLT studies were conducted on people in weight loss programs. People who worked on the treadmill and combined RLT therapy were seen to have positive changes in cellulite reduction and thigh circumference compared to those who only worked on a treadmill and did not employ RLT. These studies demonstrated that exercises and balanced nutrition combined with RLT therapy produced significantly better outcomes than exercises. Also, RLT therapy played an essential role in improving body aesthetics.

Tighter thighs and hips - Red-light therapy was also found to be effective for contouring hips and thighs. People who were exposed to RLT therapy found a reduction of 2.99 inches in overall body size. Also, researchers observed size reduction in the areas of the hips and thighs of participants. Numerous other studies demonstrate the ability of RLT to trigger lipolysis, which is the breakdown of fats and lipids in the subcutaneous fat layers of the body resulting in fat loss in targeted areas like thighs and hips.

Smaller waistline and girth - Red-light therapy research studies show an excellent tool for body contouring. Participants were exposed to red-light therapy, achieved a significant reduction in the size of their waistlines and girth.

Improved muscle repair and recovery - Research on red-light therapy has thrown up ample promise in muscle repair and recovery when used both for post- and pre-workout sessions. RLT has proven to reduce the loss of muscle strength, decrease muscle soreness, and lesser motion impairments, with effects lasting for up to 4 days after hectic workout sessions. RLT is also known to reduce knee muscle fatigue before and after exercise.

Red-light therapy for weight and fat loss is generally conducted in a fasted state for optimal outcomes. An exercise regimen suited to your weight management needs following the RLT session is known to obtain the best weight and fat loss results.

There is little doubt that red-light therapy is an effective mechanism for weight management and fat loss, especially considering the ability of red-light to completely disperse lipids and fat cells from the subcutaneous layers of the skin. Thanks to the revolutionary research findings, manufacturers have developed home-use RLT devices that help you control and manage focus and exposure time on specific targeted areas from which you wish to lose fat.

These studies also prove that RLT is a safe, pain-free, and non-invasive alternative to fat loss and weight management, mainly surgical and other invasive options with multiple, unpleasant, and unwanted side effects.

Red-light Therapy for Anti-Aging

Red-light therapy is one of the most effective and naturally available tools to improve skin health, complexion and keep aging and its unpleasant effects at bay. Numerous peer-reviewed research studies have proven multiple benefits of RLT on maintaining skin and body healthy and youthful.

RLT consists of safe and concentrated wavelengths of red light being exposed to your skin. When red-light wavelengths hit your skin, a wide range of regenerative effects occurs within the skin cells and tissues. Red light penetrates deep into the skin where it is absorbed, resulting in the stimulation of the production of elastin, collagen, and fibroblasts, all three of which are vital components for healthy, youthful-looking skin.

RLT also enhances blood circulation, which means your skin cells and tissues get increased nutrients and oxygen. Here are some of the ways that RLT promotes skin health and prevents aging:

Reduces inflammation - The anti-inflammatory effects of red-light therapy have been proven by numerous research studies. RLT has shown its efficacy for effectively managing acute and chronic inflammation so that your skin can rejuvenate and heal faster.

Increases natural collagen - Natural collagen is one of the most vital components for healthy skin. Even the best substitutes available in creams and gels are of no good compared to the natural ones.

Collagen is the most abundant protein found in the human body and is critical for the health of skin and bones. Collagen is that protein that holds everything together in our bodies, and therefore, the more naturally-formed collagen your body has, the healthier you will be.

People exposed to RLT therapy have shown increased natural collagen levels in their skin, resulting in youthful and tight skin all over the body. Also, RLT is known to increase collagen density.

Reduces fine lines and wrinkles - Red-light therapy increases the skin's moisture content, reducing fine lines and wrinkles. RLT enhances skin tone and texture, producing an overall youthful profile. People treated with RLT reported improved skin tone and texture and said their skin looked and felt better. Consequently, with RLT, your skin gets a clearer complexion and more youthful appearance than before.

Red-light therapy has also proven to help reduce and even eliminate eye wrinkles by promoting regeneration of skin cells and enhancing moisture content reduction in wrinkles around the eye.

Faster and better healing of wounds, burns, and scars - Red-light therapy has reduced the appearance of scars and improved the healing of wounds and burns significantly. RLT studies have shown that red light promotes tissue repair and recovery, which helps quick and efficient healing of wounds and their subsequent scars. Moreover, RLT is a pain-free treatment enhancing its attraction as an effective skin rejuvenating mechanism.

Reduces effects of sunburns - Excessive exposure to sunlight can potentially damage the quality of our skin, which results in sagging and old-looking skin with an increased number of fine lines and wrinkles. Studies were conducted to observe the effect of RLT on facial sunburn damage. Many of these studies proved that subjects treated with RLT for sunburns reported improved skin tone and facial skin smoothness, especially around the eyes.

Reduces acne - Researchers found that RLT is an effective acne treatment. Specifically, researchers noted that red and near-infrared light affects sebum production, one of the major contributors to acne. RLT helped to decrease the production of sebum, which, in turn, reduced acne formation. RLT is also known to control and regulate the production of cytokines, an element that impacts skin inflammation.

RLT rejuvenates the skin. Numerous studies have demonstrated that RLT is highly effective for skin regeneration and excellent for healing and reducing inflammation. It is important to note that not all kinds of red-light offer performance-boosting effects on your skin. The red light of two particular wavelengths is known to offer an optimal biological response for anti-aging and skin improvement therapy. According to RLT and dermatology experts, these two red-light wavelengths include 660 nanometers and 850 nanometers.

The red light of 660 nanometers wavelength is absorbed by the skin quickly and is, therefore, beneficial for cosmetic treatments. The red-light of 850 nanometers wavelength takes time to penetrate deeper into the skin and is, therefore, practical for pain management and other medical-related therapies.

Thanks to advanced technology, RLT is available to you in multiple forms. You can visit your dermatologist, a local spa, or a gym that provides various red-light therapy options. You can get access to full-body panels that cover your entire body or small devices designed to target one particular spot on your body. Also, home-use devices in the form of handheld machines, red-light face masks, or even highly sophisticated RLT beds are available in the market for your home use.

So, the verdict is out regarding the efficacy of RLT as an effective anti-aging therapeutic tool. It improves skin texture and tone while reducing wrinkles and fine lines. It is an anti-inflammatory therapy and helps to reduce acne, scars, and burn wounds.

Chapter 6: Is RTL Considered Safe?

The next question that many people are going to have when it comes to working with red-light therapy is whether it is safe to use or not. There is some worry that this will be strange or that it will be so strong that something can go wrong. When we look at all of the things that it can do, it is easy to see why there could be some worries about the safety of using this therapy.

Remember that this is not some strange method that will shock you or something powerful that you need to be worried about. It uses light. As the light from the sun can help improve your mood because it provides you with vitamin D, red-light therapy will be just light that comes in at a frequency that helps you get a lot of health benefits. It is as simple as that!

Unlike many of the different surgical treatments or drug treatments offered in the medical world today, red-light therapy is safe and low on side effects. Many surgeries and medications come with a massive list of side effects that are at least adverse if not fatal in some cases.

We have all seen those commercials that go through and list out all of the adverse side effects of the recommended medications. They promise to give you great results, but you have to worry about the harmful side effects. And in some cases, these side effects are going to be so bad; it is easy to wonder if it is worth your time to take the medication or live with the disease or the pain.

But with red-light therapy, you will find very few adverse side effects, and most people experience nothing terrible at all. Compared to some other methods, red-light therapy is seen as one of the most effective and safest treatments.

According to Dr. Michael Hamblin, a professor, and scientist from Harvard, "In terms of side effects, there are very few side effects. I've occasionally heard of people who put light on their head – I think one person had a headache, and a few people felt excessively sleepy."

These side effects are hardly anything to worry about. You may have a slight headache as you adjust to the detoxification, etc., of working with the light therapy, and you may need to take a nap when the treatment is done if it makes you a bit sleepy, but that is it! It is out of hundreds of studies and research done on lots of participants, and most didn't experience them at all.

You may not have time to read through all the different abstracts on the studies that have been done on red-light therapies, but with the research in this guidebook and with other books as well, you will find that there are no adverse side effects in most of the patients who went through these studies.

You will not read about many people doing red-light therapy and experiencing adverse side effects because the energy intensity from the red-light wavelengths will be below. The amount of exposure you will get from the red-light power will be so low that your tissue temperature will only increase by about a tenth of a degree overall.

It is hardly any temperature rise, and that is going to be great news. It will never cause any burns or thermal injury to the body, so you can use the light therapy even over long periods and not worry about any damage to the body due to the light.

You will also find that the devices you use for near-infrared and red-light therapy will emit a small amount of light. Most of the time, the device will emit as low as 12 watts of light. Even with this low amount (a lightbulb for your home lighting is often going to be 70 watts or more), you will see that there are some remarkably potent effects on the body.

As discussed, you will find that this kind of therapy will have pretty much no thermal effects on the body; it is a great option to use when you have a fresh injury that you want to work on healing. These injuries will be more sensitive to heat, so you do not want to work with therapies that rely on heat.

Instead, they need some therapy that is low on heat. The higher heat will irritate the injury and make the inflammation and the swelling harder to work with and worse. These heat sources could make the pain worse in the process. But with red-light therapy, you will find that it is safe to use even on these heat-sensitive injuries since there is no worry about heat.

And finally, if you are still worried that red-light therapy is not safe to use, it is an FDA-approved therapy for a couple of different health conditions. The US Government considers this kind of therapy safe for most people.

While it is still a good idea to talk to your doctor before you decide to rely solely on red-light therapy for your treatment needs, it is generally seen as safe. It can work with a variety of different health conditions, and it is going to help you see some great results in the process. And since it is easy to use, you are sure to be able to find a practitioner in your area who knows how to use the therapy, who can answer your questions about the treatment, and who can help you to go through your first (or hundredth), red-light therapy treatment.

Chapter 7: Is It Possible to Use Some Devices at Home?

Now that we know more about red-light therapy and why it is such an excellent treatment for different health conditions, it is time to learn some of the steps to get the most out of the therapy.

This section will discuss the five things you need to consider when ready to do your red-light therapy. It includes: Finding the right space for doing the treatment, the correct body position, the position of the light, the number of times you should do the sessions, and how long the sessions should last.

One thing to remember before we start with the first part is that simplicity is vital. This treatment is meant to make your life a bit easier. It is not meant to make you feel like there are a lot of particulars to remember, and you should not feel like you have to guess yourself second all of the time. The one rule to remember and that you want to follow is that you need to make things as simple as possible. It helps to make the therapy sessions more efficient and enjoyable.

So now that we have that out of the way, it is time to look at how you can create an excellent space to do these treatments. Think of it this way: If you had to start each session by carrying the device up to three flights of stairs, then plug it in and lay down on a cold hard cement floor for fifteen minutes or more, how likely would you be to keep doing the treatment, even if it did provide results?

Hopefully, the space you pick out for doing the therapy is not this bad, but it is a good illustration of what you can do to see the importance of working with a designated space for treatment. If you cannot make these sessions as pleasurable and simple as possible, you are most likely not to stick with doing the sessions for any length of time. And the more work you have to do and the more uncomfortable these sessions are, the more likely you will only do the treatment a few times before giving up in exasperation.

It is a good idea to create some place in your office or home dedicated to this light therapy treatment. It will be essential for you to get the best results when you are working with this session. And the space that you pick needs to make the treatment itself as simple and as pleasurable as possible.

Now, you will be able to set this up in any manner that you would like. You may find that working with a yoga mat, a blanket, or even a towel spread out on the floor where you need to lay or sit down on can make it more comfortable. Adding a pillow or two can be great as well. And, some people find that it is best to lay on a bed or a cot to add a bit more comfort to the situation.

In addition to the above options for comfort, you may decide to keep a timer in place. Some patients like to just use the timer on their phone for this, which is fine. But if you want to work with a designated timer just for the red-light therapy, then make sure that you leave it in the treatment space. It saves time and effort from constantly having to look for it later.

Another consideration when picking out a space for your treatments is that there should be some power outlet nearby. Your light device has to stay plugged in at all times during the therapy, and if it can recharge in between sessions, this can make things a bit easier.

From there, you may think about what else you would like to have in your treatment space. It is your unique space, and it will hopefully be set up to help you relax and stay focused during the session. Each person is going to bring in different things to the mix, and this is fine. But you may want to consider what would make you the most comfortable and relaxed and help you gain the proper focus when working through light therapy.

With the space in mind, also consider when you would like to do the light therapy. It is often recommended that you do it either in the morning or in the evening. You can choose the period that works best for you. Both of these are valuable times, and you have to go with one that is either going to help energize you for the morning or give you some repair in the evening after a hard day.

For example, some people find that doing therapy in the morning is best for them. The red-light treatment is going to help you to be more energized and ready for the day. It can add more focus, improve memory, repair the cells and help you to detoxify your body before you get out for the day. Depending on the kind of condition you are dealing with, you may find that the morning treatment timing will be more efficient for you in the process.

But then some benefits come with doing the light treatments in the evening. It is an excellent way to repair any damage that happens to your cells during the day. It can relieve some of the headaches, stress, and more built up throughout your daily life. This one works well if you suffer from anxiety and other conditions that make it hard to fall asleep at night.

The main point of this section is that we need to have a good space for treatment and choose the time that works best for us. Your goal, if you have the room to make it happen, is to have a designated space that is just for this therapy, but try to at least get something that is going to be comfortable and will allow you to focus and relax while the red-light therapy is doing its work.

The Body Position During the Red-light Therapy

We took some time looking at the best places to set up your treatments to help you be relaxed, comfortable and focused on the session. Now we will move on to the second part of this, which is the body position. The way you will position the body when you do one of the treatment sessions will matter. Suppose you have your body placed in some position uncomfortably, and you cannot relax all the way. In that case, it will not take long before this stops holding your interest, and you decide not to use the device and get its benefits any longer.

Remember that we are going to be more motivated to do things that we find pleasant and rewarding. It is why we need to make sure that we find a position for the body that is comfortable and still gives us a chance to relax all the way, or we will stop. The good news is there are three options that you can use when it comes to how to position your body while still getting the full benefits of the red-light therapy. The three methods that you can use include lying down, sitting, and standing.

The Standing Body Position

A few devices for red-light therapy are designed to help those who plan to stand up for their whole session. These can include some LED light panels held with a stand or placed on the wall

While the idea of standing up for your treatment may seem like a good idea to try, do you want to stand stuck in one place for a possible 20 minutes two times a day, depending on your treatment? Standing in one spot for an extended period can be uncomfortable because of the weight of supporting your body. And it may be challenging for you to fully relax and be as comfortable as you need to see the results.

If this is what you are the most comfortable with using during the treatment or what works the best for the space you are in, then go ahead and use it. But for most people, it is not going to be comfortable. And you may find that standing still for that long can add in more discomfort than what you were trying to fix with the light therapy. It is why most people would prefer working with the other two body positions.

The Sitting Body Position

The second option that you can work with is the sitting body position. If you can sit in a comfortable recliner or a sofa, you can relax and enjoy the treatment. There are a lot of benefits of working with this because it will be more comfortable than standing for the treatment duration, and you get some options for where to sit.

But there are still many people looking to go with another position because some disadvantages come with this method. Some of the main downsides that come with the seated position include some of the following:

When you do the therapy while sitting, you need to have some supportive muscles to help you contract, preventing you from getting into total relaxation.

When you do the therapy while sitting, it can make it a bit harder to position the red light so that you can get a total amount of healing.

When you do the therapy while sitting, it is sometimes uncomfortable, and sometimes people may find it a bit painful during the treatment.

There are a lot of benefits to sitting during the therapy, and it is a much better option than standing. It is a lot more comfortable to work with and can make it easier to relax and benefit. But, there are still some disadvantages, so you will have to compare to see if this method works for you to reap the full benefits of the red-light therapy treatment.

The Laying Down Body Position

If you can do this, then laying down is going to be the best option to choose. It is seen as the gold standard for red-light therapy treatment sessions. Laying down is going to give you all of the comforts that you are looking for. It makes it easier to relax every muscle in your body, and it is the only position out of the three that is the safest if you fall asleep during the treatment.

In many centers offering this therapy, the devices will be hung from the ceiling, with the patient lying on a massage therapy table under that light. It is one way to do it. Finding an above supportive structure from which you can hang the light can require some creativity, but it is something to try.

It can be a bit harder to work with for some people, but if you are trying to place it on your leg, stomach, or somewhere similar, it is possible to just lay it down on that area. It will not cause burns or any other issues, so you will be safe using it in this manner. You can then relax as the body enjoys the red-light therapy and all it can provide to you.

The Position of the Light During Treatment

The next thing we need to look at when we are doing one of our treatments is the position of the light. Since you will find that laying down will be the ideal body position when you do your treatment, most of the attention that we focus on here will be with where the light needs to be while you are lying down. But first, we can talk about where to put the light when you are either sitting or standing.

First, you can choose to do light therapy while standing. When standing for the treatment, the position of your light can be on a vertical stand, or you can use a light that is mounted onto a wall near you. It will be beneficial because you can get the therapy without holding onto the light during the session. However, there is a disadvantage in that you will have to stand up during the treatment to get the benefits.

Then, you have the choice of sitting while doing the light therapy. It is a good option, and the location for the light can be on a table right in front of you, or you can place it on your lap facing you. The light position here will make it more difficult to treat any body part that is not the face or the chest area since the distance is nearer for those areas when you choose this.

You can also pick some different lighting positions when you are lying down. Compared to the sitting or standing position, you will find that positioning the light for laying down will be easier. You can lay down in the correct position and then place the device right beside you on the floor or the bed, aiming that light at the part of the body that needs to have the treatment.

You can also choose to hang the light device from something above you if this seems like it is the best choice to use. But for most people, laying down and facing the light in the direction of the part of the body that needs the treatment will be the best, and often the easiest, place to put the light.

If you need to work on pain in your lower back, you can place the light behind you right against the area causing the pain and then relax. If you have a sore knee, lay down with the light against the knee. It is the same no matter what part of the body you feel pain or issues with, no matter what kind of treatment you want to work with. Just lay the red light against that body part while you relax and enjoy the light coming in a while laying down.

As we mentioned before, laying down will be the ideal body position when doing your red-light therapy. It will afford you a lot of comforts while being safe and still making light positioning easier. It is the simplicity you need, as we talked about before, and it ensures that you can relax, which is required when you want to get the most out of the session.

Chapter 8: Instructions on How Long to Use the Infrared Therapy For

The Duration of the Session

The fourth thing that we need to spend some time looking through when we want to do some red-light therapy is the duration of the session. It means that most people need to consider how long they want to use the red light each time they begin treatment. The number of times you do it during the day and the duration of the sessions depends on the problem you are trying to solve and how bad that issue is from the beginning.

The session's duration will be the number of minutes you expose a body part to the red-light session. You may find that experimenting a bit and seeing what works the best for you will help you get the most efficient amount of time for each session.

Science has been determined the amount of time for a session to get the best results. It depends on the condition you are dealing with. It is also important to remember that nothing is set in stone. You may have to go for a bit longer, but then there is a chance you will need less time to see results. Starting at the base discussed in various studies is an excellent place to look at, but you can add or take away time-based on what works for you.

If you are worried about going for too long with the therapy, starting with more minor or shorter sessions is acceptable and then building up to what you want. But remember that red-light therapy will be one of the safest therapies and treatments that you can do for most ailments, so there isn't much to worry about when you go for the length of time you have chosen for this treatment.

The first thing you may consider doing with this treatment is to do the red light on the whole body. If you feel comfortable doing this, you can lie in a fetal position without any clothes on and with the light facing a position right between the chest and stomach. It may sound awkward, but remember that you are alone and that this will be an excellent way to prepare your body and get some overall healing right from the beginning.

The goal of the full body treatment is that it is going to help you to reach as many of the cells in your body as you can. From this position, if you do it the right way, you should get the upper arms, the chest, the stomach, and the upper legs in one shot. It is excellent if you only have one light and want to work on as much of your body as possible in one treatment session.

Even if you bought the light to help with a particular part of the body, such as your chronic pain or an injured ankle, it is still a good idea to work on the whole body before moving on to working with just that body part. It is one way for you to see the healing power that even a tiny device for red-light therapy can do for your body.

When you decide to work with the complete body treatment, you will notice that you feel better in no time. It is because you are working on as many of the cells in the body as possible. You may start to notice that you feel better, less depressed and that other things are healed – something that you may not have even seen was bothering you previously. If you decide to do this kind of treatment, working on this session for about 20 minutes is a good start.

For most people, working with the treatment for 15 to 20 minutes is enough time to get the results that you want. But you may need to experiment with this for a bit. While there is no harm with going for a bit longer on your treatment if you choose because all it will do is improve your health without any adverse side effects, most people like to find the timing of the session that works for them.

You can have two choices with this: You can start with the 20 minutes for the treatment, or you can go through and slowly increase the time until you reach the one that seems to provide you with the most benefits. This one takes a bit longer but lets you know the personalized time for the red-light treatment that works the best for the disease or disorder you are dealing with.

For example, you may start with a treatment that is five minutes long and see how that does. You may then notice that this is not long enough to provide you with all of the relief you want, so you up to your sessions to ten minutes a day and see how that works for you. Then you add on 15 minutes, and then 20 minutes, and so on.

You may find that you are good at 15 minutes and don't feel like there is much difference between 15 minutes to 20 minutes. Then this means that you can pick between the two and go with the period that is the best for you. Once you start feeling that the benefits are not getting any stronger or better when you go up in time, this is a good sign that the lowest time frame where you started feeling this way will be the right one for you.

In addition, you may find that each part of your body may need to have a different session duration. After ten minutes, you may feel relief from an ankle problem but find that you need closer to 20 or 25 minutes to help the stress or anxiety in your life. It is perfectly normal, and taking the time to experiment will make it easier to find the time frames that work best for you.

The session duration that you choose is an important consideration to think about ahead of time. Whether you decide to go with the standard timings for your condition or are willing to mess around a bit and see which method works the best for you, you will find that the red-light therapy will provide you with the benefits you need. You have to identify how long of a session you need to do to get those great benefits.

The Frequency of the Sessions You Do with Red-light

The fifth thing that we need to consider when we are getting ready to work with our session is the frequency of the sessions. We have to determine how often we will do these sessions: Whether it is a few times a day, a few times a week, or just at any time we feel the problem is flaring up again.

The session frequency will be defined as the number of treatment sessions you need to go through each day or week. Studies have shown that going between two and twenty sessions per week will be effective as a general guideline and considering what works for you. It means that you may need to get between two and three sessions a day for the treatment, although some people are just fine if they do one or two sessions spread out throughout the week.

However, you can choose the number of times that will work for you. There shouldn't be any worries about how many times you use the device, and if you want to experiment with this and use it more often than two or three times weekly, this is fine because red-light therapy is safe and will not cause any harm with more use.

For many people, at least, starting with two treatments a day will work well. It helps to fix the cells and keeps them as healthy as possible. Over time, they may decide to go up or down on the number of sessions done based on their feelings. Doing one when you wake up in the morning to energize and prepare you for the day, and then doing one at night to help you get a more restful and peaceful sleep can be the best options for your needs.

One question that is often asked here is that, since the red light can energize the cells inside our bodies, do we need to worry about doing the treatment at night, and how could it interrupt the patient's sleep? Put your mind at ease here because the answer is no, and many patients have found that doing a therapy session before they go to bed can help them fall asleep and stay asleep better at night.

The reason for this is that the red light will reduce both the adrenaline and cortisol levels in the body, which is essential to help them fall asleep at night. In addition, since the red-light therapy can help us reduce the amount of stress we are dealing with, it is even easier to fall asleep.

Of course, before you start to make some changes to what you are doing with your red-light therapy treatments, take some time to try it out beforehand. It works with all of the tips that we have looked at when it comes to the session. Figure out what position it should be in, where the light should go, how often you should do the sessions, and even the number of times you should do the sessions. This red-light therapy treatment is meant to work well for you, and taking the time to personalize it and make it fit in with your comfort level is crucial if you want to see results.

Common Mistakes People Make When Using Red-light Therapy

When it comes to using red-light therapy, you will find that there are a lot of great benefits that you are going to be getting: You can increase the density of your bones, help with weight loss, reduce anxiety and depression, learn how to reduce stress levels, and so much more. As more research is done about this therapy, almost everyone will likely use the treatment to repair their health and make them feel so much better.

It is also essential to know some common mistakes you need to know using red-light therapy. It would help if you learned how to avoid some of these common mistakes to ensure that you will get the most out of your treatments and not feel like the treatment is not working for your needs or your particular health conditions. Some of the most common mistakes that beginners may make when they first decide to work with the red-light therapy treatments for their health will include the following:

They Don't Do It for Long Enough

Timing your light therapy sessions is crucial. If you don't spend enough time under the light each day, you may not get the full benefits that you are looking for. It is essential to experiment and figure out how long the red light works best for your condition. Some people may do ten minutes a few times a day, and others will need closer to 20 or more minutes to get the same results. Each person will be different, and it will be determined by how your body responds to the light.

If you try out the therapy a few times and don't feel like it is doing anything for you, it is time to experiment a little bit. Try a few different methods to see which one seems to provide you with the relief you need. By adding just five minutes to your session, you may find that you can go from not feeling anything to feeling fabulous in no time!

They Didn't Do Their Research

Doing your research about red-light therapy will make a big difference in your outlook on it and how much you will be able to use it. Whether you need some scientific information to figure out if this treatment is effective or not, or you are interested in learning how this treatment will benefit your health, you will find that there are many studies and more on this.

The worst thing about having this lack of research is that people do not know all the incredible health benefits they can reap. They may have heard about a handful of the health benefits that come with red-light therapy, but because they haven't done all of the research, they don't realize that they can improve their health condition from it. The more you learn about red-light therapy, the more you can see that the treatment can help to benefit anyone who decides to use it.

If you have gone through this guidebook and have not found the condition you need to fix, this doesn't mean that all hope is lost.

It simply means that you need to find the research that points out how great this treatment can be for everyone.

They Are Skeptical About the Process

We have been trained well by the big pharmaceuticals and others who make a lot of money in our world of medicine. We learn that we are supposed to take expensive medications, do costly surgeries, and sacrifice our health to make sure that we can get rid of some disease or illness. It is big business for some companies, but it is not always the best choice for us.

All the information that we have been fed is not in our best interests, but it makes us skeptical about some other treatments that work but don't seem to fit in with what traditional medicine tells us about. It makes it hard because many people miss out on some of the benefits of this kind of treatment, as they don't think it can work for them or anyone else.

But there are so many great benefits that come with the use of red-light therapy. And it can benefit pretty much anyone willing to give it a try. Even if you are a big fan of medicine, surgery, and the conventional medical things that we use now, why not give it a try? There are no adverse side effects, and just because red-light therapy is used, it doesn't mean that you have to give up on the other stuff entirely. But why not enhance those a bit? Even if you don't think it works, there are no side effects, and it could be what you are looking for.

They Don't Learn How to Relax All of the Ways

You need to focus here because you need to relax while the red-light therapy is doing its job. It may sound like not that big of a deal, but you do want to make sure that you are not tensed up and that the body and the mind can relax for the total duration of the therapy, whether it is 15 minutes 20 minutes, or even half an hour or more to get the results.

It may be hard for some people to do. But it is hard for you to get results from any therapy that you try, in any type of treatment that you try out. Being tense slows down the process, and you will not get the relief you would like.

There are a few steps that you can take that will make it easier to relax. If you need to take a few minutes to do some deep breathing exercises before starting, doing some reading or even taking a nice bath can help. You may find that a few minutes of meditation will make a difference. You will see a massive difference between doing a session while tensed up and worried and when you do one after finding a method that relaxes you before starting.

Not Choosing the Right Device

The next thing you need to focus on with this therapy is picking out a device that will provide you with the necessary treatment. You do not want to pick out a device that is not red or infrared technology, or it will not do the promised work.

It is where you need to be able to do some research ahead of time. There are some high-quality options for devices on the market, but many companies are trying to jump on the bandwagon, which may not offer you the excellent product you are looking for.

Chapter 9: Top 10 Proven Benefits of Red Light

Now that you've seen the long list of diseases and conditions that red and near-infrared-light therapy can benefit from let's go a little more in-depth into some of them. The findings of some of these studies are remarkable, and they will give you a good indication of how powerful a remedy red-light is and what it can do for you.

Here is my top 10 list of some of the most common ailments that can be effectively treated using red and near-infrared-light therapies.

1. Melt Your Belly Fat

According to the Centre for Disease Control (CDC), more than one-third (36.5%) of U.S. adults are obese. Obese people have an increased risk of many conditions, including heart disease, stroke, type 2 diabetes, and cancer, so correcting this condition is vital for long-term health.

Another benefit of fat reduction in an obese person is the money saved on medical costs every year. How much money? The medical prices for people who have obesity are $1,429 higher per year than those of 'normal' weight.[1]

So there you have it – reducing obesity can not only improve the health of the individual, but it can reduce their cost of living and the stress associated with having to spend more money on medical bills.

There are no shortages of people, programs, and devices claiming they can help people burn fat – but we all know many of them turn out to be fraudulent and don't work. Others can help you lose weight, but they do so in excessively stressful and unhealthy ways.

The results?

Remarkably, the women who received the near-infrared-light therapy following exercise *doubled* the amount of fat loss compared to exercise alone. Additionally, the women in the training + phototherapy group reported a more significant increase in skeletal muscle mass than the placebo group.

Other studies have reported similar findings in obese people who combined exercise with red-light therapy. Still, even studies that *did not* include training have reported significant fat reduction from red-light therapy alone.

Scientists from George Washington University conducted an independent physician-led trial in 2013 to test the ability of red laser light (635nm) to reduce fat on the waist, hips, and thighs of obese individuals. Laser treatments were administered to 8 obese patients and consisted of 20-minute sessions every second day for two weeks. The results were remarkable when researchers assessed the patients three weeks after the trial began (one week after treatments ended). "Compared with baseline, a statistically significant 2.99 in. (7.59 cm) mean loss was observed at the post-procedure evaluation point (P < 0.0001)."

Translation: Patients lost 3 inches of fat in just two weeks of red-light therapy treatment.

2. Accelerate Wound Healing

Whether it's from an accident during physical activity or chemical pollutants in our food and environment, we all sustain injuries regularly. Anything that can help accelerate the body's innate healing process will free up resources and focus its available energy reserves on maintaining optimal health.

Dr. Harry Whelan from the Medical College of Wisconsin has studied red-light in cell cultures and humans for decades. His work in the laboratory has shown that skin and muscle cells grown in cultures and exposed to LED infrared light grow 150-200% faster than control cultures not stimulated by the light.

Working with Naval doctors in Norfolk, Virginia, and San Diego, California, to treat injured soldiers, Dr. Whelan and his team found that musculoskeletal training injuries treated with the light-emitting diodes improved by 40%.

In 2014, a group of scientists from three universities in Brazil conducted a scientific review of the effects of red-light on wound healing. After reviewing a total of 68 studies, most of which were conducted on animals using wavelengths ranging from 632 to 830 nm, the study concluded: "…phototherapy, either by LASER or LED, is an effective therapeutic modality to promote healing of skin wounds."

No matter how you have been wounded, red-light therapy can be used as a non-tissue-specific healing accelerant.

3. Increase Bone Density

Bone density and the ability of the body to build new bone are essential for people recovering from injuries. It's also crucial for older people since our bones tend to become weaker with age progressively. Anybody who isn't sick and wants to remain physically active for as much of their lives as possible has an interest in building and maintaining strong, healthy bones.

The bone-healing benefits of red and near-infrared light have been demonstrated in many laboratory studies.

In 2013, researchers from São Paulo, Brazil, studied the effects of red and near-infrared light on the healing of rat bones. First, a piece of bone was sliced off the upper leg (osteotomy) of 45 rats, which were then split into three groups: Group 1 received no light, group 2 was administered red-light (660-690nm), and group 3 was exposed to near-infrared-light (790-830nm).

The study found "a significant increase in the degree of mineralization (gray level) in both groups treated with the laser after seven days" and interestingly, "after 14 days, only the group treated with laser therapy in the infrared spectrum showed higher bone density."

Here are a few more studies on light therapy for bone health and their conclusions.

2003 study conclusion: "We conclude that LLLT had a positive effect on the repair of bone defects implanted with inorganic bovine bone."

2006 study conclusion: "The results of studies indicate that bone irradiated mostly with infrared (IR) wavelengths shows increased osteoblastic proliferation, collagen deposition, and bone neoformation when compared to nonirradiated bone."

2008 study conclusion: "The use of laser technology has been used to improve the clinical results of bone surgeries and to promote a more comfortable postoperative period and quicker healing."13

Red and near-infrared light can be used to build more robust bones. After breaking a bone or incurring any kind of bodily injury, near-infrared and red-light therapies should be used as the first line of treatment by anybody wanting a speedy recovery.

4. Increase Testosterone

Throughout history, the essence of a man has been linked to his primary male hormone, testosterone. At around the age of 30, testosterone levels begin to decline, resulting in many negative changes to a man's physical and mental health and wellbeing: Reduced sexual function, low energy levels, reduced muscle mass, and increased fat, among others.

When you factor in the endless environmental contaminants, stress, and poor nutrition that are so common today, it's no surprise that we are seeing an epidemic of low testosterone in men the world over.

At the end of the 5-day trial, while untreated rats had no increase in testosterone, rats exposed to one 30-minute light therapy treatment per day had significantly elevated testosterone levels. "…Serum T level was significantly increased in the 808nm wavelength group. In the 670 nm wavelength group, serum T level was also significantly increased at the same intensity of 360 J/cm2/day," concluded researchers.

For this same reason, it's essential to keep the light about a foot away when treating testicles with red-light therapy. Don't let this discourage you from experimenting. Important: if you position your red light too close and apply too much heating to the area during treatment, your sex drive and testosterone levels may be impeded for a short time before returning to baseline.

5. Enhance Brain Function

Nootropics (pronounced: no-oh-troh-picks), also called smart drugs or cognitive enhancers, have undergone a dramatic spike in popularity in recent years and are being used by many people to enhance brain functions such as memory, creativity, and motivation.

The positive effects of red light on brain function are significant and well established scientifically. Red and near-infrared light could very well be the most powerful nootropic ever discovered. Let's look at some evidence for this.

If you're in school, red-light can help you memorize and recall information, increase your ability to work for long periods, and have your brain functioning optimally for tests.

Parents who administer red-light on the foreheads of their young children will not only help their kids learn better, but it will allow them to connect with other students and develop long-lasting relationships more easily. I'm excited to see the geniuses that arise in this world directly resulting from being raised by parents who regularly applied red-light to their brains and bodies.

6. Eliminate Anxiety and Depression

Depression affects 121 million people worldwide, and that's only the number of people *officially* diagnosed with it. The truth is we all experience depression at some point in our lives. And when we do, many of us turn to drugs or other drug-like behaviors that help raise dopamine levels, such as pornography, social media, or video games. I know that many people long to feel the liberation associated with not having to depend on these props to cope with life.

University students: - "the ones who are supposed to be our smartest and healthiest leaders-of-tomorrow" – experience significantly higher rates of depression than your average population, according to a 2012 scientific review.

Even more troubling: "Depression is associated with high suicidality," wrote scientist M.S. Reddy in 2010. "About 50% of individuals who have committed suicide carried a primary diagnosis of depression," continued Reddy.

Anxiety is even more common than depression – it's the most common mental illness in the U.S. – affecting 40 million adults age 18 and older (18.1%).

Existing medical treatments for anxiety and depression are toxic, tend to numb people out, and have even been implicated in causing aggressive and suicidal behavior. It is primarily due to a misunderstanding of the role of serotonin in the human body. However, that is a subject for another time as it's beyond the scope of this book. New and effective therapies are desperately needed to curb anxiety, depression, and today's alarming rate of suicide.

Just imagine how much better life would be for us all if people had a way of melting away their feelings of anxiety and depression.

Can red-light therapy treat anxiety and depression?

In 2009, a group of scientists from Harvard University tested the effects of near-infrared light on ten subjects with major depression. Researchers applied the light directly to the forehead of patients in one 16-minute session. After just one treatment with near-infrared light, "Patients experienced highly significant reductions in both HAM-D [depression] and HAM-A [anxiety] scores following treatment, with the greatest reductions occurring at two weeks."

Translation: Near-infrared-light therapy resulted in long-lasting reductions in depression and anxiety from *just one* treatment.

7. Eliminate Acne Vulgaris

Acne is the most widespread skin condition in the U.S., affecting up to 50 million Americans annually.

People react differently to acne on their face and body, but it often results in poor self-image, depression, anxiety, and many times permanent physical scarring of the skin.

A 2001 experiment from Queens Medical Center in Nottingham, UK, found that acne was prevalent in 50% of adolescents and had a "considerable impact on emotional health in this age group."

Towards the end of grade school, I began developing pretty severe acne. I remember how much it affected me psychologically. In reality, it wasn't nearly as bad physically as I perceived it to be, but I can remember seeing a cute girl in class or the halls, and all that was on my mind was that I needed to make sure she didn't see me it. It harmed my relationships and social interaction, and I wish I had something better than the ineffective cream the dermatologist gave me to treat it.

Can light therapy treat acne?

Iranian scientists compared the effects of red (630nm) and near-infrared (890nm) laser therapy on 28 patients with facial acne in 2012. Participants in the study were given light therapy on their face 2-times per week for six weeks, and their skin conditions were then assessed.

Ten weeks after treatment, acne lesions were *significantly decreased in those treated with the red light*, but the decrease wasn't signed with the near-infrared light.

Thanks to the scientific discovery of red light as a remedy for acne, present and future generations of children no longer have to deal with swollen, red, painful pus-oozing pimples and all the negative implications on their psychology and social lives.

It is your duty and mine to make kids aware of red-light therapy as a safe and effective remedy for acne, so they know where to reach if and when pimples begin to form.

8. Relieve Pain

America is a nation in pain, according to a 2015 study by researchers at the National Institutes of Health. How much pain?

Nearly 50 million American adults (11.2%) reported experiencing pain daily for the previous three months.

Some of the most common pain medications that people reach for when feeling pain are Tylenol, Ibuprofen, or other drugs classified as Non-Steroidal Anti-Inflammatory Drugs (NSAIDS). Interestingly, these common painkillers have been shown to cause heart attacks, strokes, and cancer, except aspirin, which reduces the risk of these same complications. In 2015, the FDA issued a strong warning that all NSAIDs except aspirin can trigger heart attacks and strokes.

In other words, people experiencing pain are using medications that are slowly killing them. Interestingly, aspirin and red-light kill pain in similar ways by reducing an enzyme called COX-2. More about that later. We know that safer and more effective treatments are needed to reduce the chronic pain people are experiencing.

Here are the conclusions of a few recent publications on pain reduction using therapeutic red and near-infrared light:

A 2006 systematic review:

"There is strong evidence that LLLT [low-level laser therapy] modulates the inflammatory process and relieves acute pain in the short-term."

A 2009 systematic review published in *The Lancet*:

"We show that LLLT reduces pain immediately after treatment in acute neck pain and up to 22 weeks after completion of treatment in patients with chronic neck pain."

A 2014 review:

"[red and near-infrared] Laser causes pain relief without any side effects."

9. Regrow Hair on a Balding Scalp

Hair loss (alopecia) is a pervasive disorder affecting more than 50% of the worldwide population.

In the United States, an estimated 35 million men and 21 million women suffer from some form of hair loss, and around 40% of men will have noticeable hair loss by the age of 35.

If you think of each hair follicle as a hair-producing factory, it can be said that in somebody experiencing hair loss, the factory has been shut down. If those unhealthy follicles can be healed, then, in theory, they can once again produce hair.

 "I only have to venture to a major street in San Francisco to find that if there were an 'effective' treatment for baldness, a majority of men are either not aware of it or are choosing to be bald," wrote hair-loss researcher Danny Roddy.

Can red-light help regrow hair on a balding scalp?

American and Hungarian researchers conducted a review in 2014 of studies involving hair loss treatment with red and near-infrared laser therapy. The examination reports that red and near-infrared laser therapies have been demonstrated to stimulate hair growth in both mice and men and women in many controlled clinical trials. "LLLT for hair growth in both men and women appears to be both safe and effective. The optimum wavelength, coherence, and dosimetric parameters remain to be determined," they concluded.

10. Heal Arthritis

Arthritis is a crippling ailment from which many people suffer worldwide. An estimated 22.7% of US adults were diagnosed with some form of arthritis between 2013-2015. That's almost 55 million people who could benefit from an effective treatment for the condition.

I've never experienced arthritis myself, but one of my previous girlfriend's friends had arthritis severely, and remarkably she was only 28 years old at the time. Whereas arthritis used to exist almost exclusively in older people, it seems more prevalent today among young people.

The closest thing I've experienced to arthritis was after I stubbed my finger on a basketball. I remember not bending my finger for about a week due to the swelling and pain. I can hardly imagine having to deal with that immobility, pain, and discomfort regularly. I feel for anybody who has arthritis, and I added this section to the book with you in mind.

Currently, there are dozens of different FDA-approved drugs for arthritis, all of which come with limited successes as well as their own set of potentially serious side effects.

Can red-light be used to treat arthritis?

Dr. Michael R. Hamblin, a Harvard professor from the Department of Dermatology, has been experimenting with red-light for decades and is considered one of the world's leading authorities on the subject. In 2013, he published a study titled *Can Osteoarthritis Be Treated with Light?* The study tested the use of near-infrared laser light (810nm) on arthritis in rats.

Remarkably, after inducing arthritis in the rats and treating them just *one time* with the near-infrared laser, inflammation was found to be significantly reduced in just 24 hours. "A single application of LLLT produced significant reductions in inflammatory cell infiltration and inflammatory cytokines 24 hours later."

For those who've been frustrated by the struggle to find safe and effective treatment for arthritis, look no further than red-light therapy. It could change your life.

What book on red-light therapy would be complete without addressing its impact on the one disease that threatens human existence more than any other?

Chapter 10:   FAQ About Red-light Therapy

Q: My specialist (chiropractor, naturopath, etc.) said that solitary his/her laser will work, not the LED lights. Who is correct?

It is a fantasy that lone lasers have these impacts. Numerous individuals thought for a long time that solitary lasers had these impacts (since they were first discovered with laser gadgets). However, as of late, it has been demonstrated that non-laser light (like from LED devices of the suitable wavelengths) has similar impacts.

More than 250 examinations are utilizing LED red and close infrared-light treatment that has been done in simply the most recent couple of years (since it was understood that you could get indistinguishable impacts from LEDs from lasers). The investigations that think about them have found essentially similar advantages. What's more, there is essentially nothing to demonstrate that one needs lasers to create these impacts. Indeed, even a few organizations (like Thor Laser) that have been creating laser advances for quite a long time are currently delivering LED items.

As indicated by Harvard analyst Michael Hamblin, Ph.D. (broadly viewed as the world's top expert on close infrared and red-light treatment),

"The vast majority of the early work in this field was completed with different lasers. It was believed that laser light had some unique attributes not controlled by light from other light sources, for example, sunlight, fluorescent or glowing lights, and now LEDs. Anyway, every one of the investigations that have been finished contrasting lasers with identical light sources with comparative wavelength and power thickness of their discharge has found no distinction between them."

Q: Are there any worries of EMFs (electromagnetic fields) if the gadget is extremely near the body?

Every electronic gadget transmits EMFs (electromagnetic fields), and the wellbeing impacts of EMFs are still discussed. By the strictest security norms from Europe, you would prefer not to be formally presented to more than 3mG (milligauss).

If it's not too much trouble, only for reference for correlation, note that your mobile phone produces considerably more than this at regular intervals. If it's being used, it radiates undeniably more than 3mG (as much as 50mG and even near 100mG). A family unit blender transmits as much as one hundred mG.

I've measured the EMF yield of the Joovv, Red Rush360, and Platinum LED lights, and EMF yield is moderate (keeping pace with a run-of-the-mill PC or workstation, and not exactly a mobile phone) inside 0-3 inches. As you move away by 5 inches or something like that, there are no perceivable EMFs. (Note: EMFs drop off drastically as you move away from the source). So by utilizing it at any rate 6" away from your body, you can get a solid portion of light with no worry at all over EMFs. Anyplace over around 3" out will be exceptionally sheltered. However, if you need to be amazingly wary and have no EMF introduction by any stretch of the imagination, going more than 6" is perfect. It will take out your presentation to EMFs. (Note: I have just figured in this reality to my suggested treatment separations illustrated in this book by encouraging you to remain in any event 6" away, so fundamentally, the EMF issue is a non-issue since there are no perceptible EMFs at the treatment separations.)

One increasingly significant point: One should likewise consider the quality of the EMF produced, yet considerably more critically, the recurrence of the portion. What I mean is that sitting with your hands on your PC or having a cell phone on your body for a few hours every day (basic practices for a great many people in the Western world) is endless to a greater degree a worry for your wellbeing than a 3-or 15-minute presentation to the red/NIR light done once per day or each other day. In case you're going to stress over EMFs, at that point, I propose guiding your focus toward things like the mobile phone you have on your body or in your grasp for perhaps hours every day, your utilization of PCs and iPads, and so on. Those are considerably more genuine concerns.

Also, once more, without much of a stretch, you can take out the EMF worry with red/NIR lights out and out just by being at any rate 6 inches from the gadget. So this is a non-issue.

Q: What distance should the light be for the most powerful impact?

The closer the light is, the more grounded the portion. So "greatest impact" would be with the LED light essentially on your body, as close as could reasonably be expected. However, because these electronic gadgets produce EMFs (electromagnetic fields) and the wellbeing impacts of EMFs are still discussed, I prescribe limiting EMF introduction by being at any rate 3" away from the gadget. As clarified above, going in any event 6" away is perfect.

For more profound tissues, treating from 6" or 12" is perfect. For skin hostile to maturing impacts, moving the light further away to 12", 18", 24" or even 36", which is that since light spreads as you move away from the source, going further away enables you to treat a lot bigger body territories at the same time.

See the dosing area for progressively explicit guidelines on the best separations and portions for various purposes.

Q: How long and how frequently would it be advisable for me to do the red-light sessions?

The extent to do the treatment has been clarified in the area of dosing in this book. Concerning recurrence of utilization, there is no all-inclusive concurrence on the dosing recurrence in the exploration, so I can suggest depending on what is generally regular in the examination and dependent on my encounters with a massive number of individuals I've worked with. When all is said in done, I've discovered that more than once every day is excessive. For the vast majority, the ideal recurrence is 3-6x every week. (For example: between each other day or consistently). For an intense issue, such as mending damage, it might be perfect for doing one treatment for each day. (For example, You just sprained your lower leg, and you need it to recuperate as quick as would be prudent). I don't suggest accomplishing more than one treatment for each day. Recollect the biphasic portion reaction clarified before in this book. Doing an excess will give less beneficial outcomes than doing the perfect sum.

Q: Is there a best time of day to do it? Or on the other hand, are there sure suggested practices you have for utilizing the light for explicit issues?

There are scarcely any focuses worth making here:

- If you are utilizing the light for the psychological upgrade, utilizing it on your head proceeding the period you have to center or perform is likely the best approach. (For instance, in the first part of the previous day beginning your workday).
- If you utilize the light to improve execution during physical movement, use the LED on the muscles that will be a most dynamic 5-an hour before the auction.
- If you are utilizing the light to improve fat misfortune or muscle gain because of activity, utilizing it previously or

after exercise is perfect (whatever season of day that is). (Note: Some investigations use it earlier and others after. I, for one, support utilizing it after; however, a few examinations have demonstrated excellent outcomes with applying it before practice.)

- If you utilize it to speed recovery after exercise, utilizing it directly after a workout or a few hours after the fact is perfect (whatever season of day that is).

- For most purposes – for example, against maturing impacts, boosting insusceptibility, and diminishing irritation – the hour of the day likely doesn't make a difference by any means. (It is hypothetically conceivable that specific occasions may be slightly superior to other people, yet there is no exploration to show this).

- If you are utilizing it for cellulite reduction, it might be helpful to directly use the light on the influenced territory before doing exercise (whatever season of day that is).

- However, red-light doesn't influence the circadian cadence so much as different wavelengths (like blue or green light, regular indoor white house lighting, and so on). , The red light like these powerful LED lights will stifle melatonin discharge and upset rest on the off chance that you use it excessively near sleep time. So I would recommend not utilizing it inside an hour of rest. (NIR is likely substantially less of an issue than obvious red-light in such manner).

Q: Can you split into a few trim sessions for the same impact?

You can conceivably do that. However, I prescribe that individuals stay without more than one session every day for the most part. I propose doing one longer treatment instead of numerous shorter medicines.

Q: I have the light and have done a few medications. However, how would I realize that it's working? How rapidly will I see or feel the impacts?

Much like enhancements or physician-endorsed drugs, you can't generally realize simply dependent on your abstract sentiments if something is working or not. Take, for instance, a statin medicate that brings down cholesterol. Would you be able to feel that it is attempting to bring down your cholesterol? No, not. In any case, if you get your blood drawn and measure your blood lipids, you will see that it is bringing down your cholesterol.

As another model, suppose you're utilizing it for muscle addition or fat misfortune, and consider that the exploration says that as a rule, red and close infrared-light treatment increment fat misfortune or muscle gain by 30% past simply doing the activity alone. (That is an enormous impact incidentally). In any case, the distinction between you losing four crawls off your abdomen (without the light) versus 5.2 inches (with the light), you have no chance to get of realizing that the light made you lose an extra 1.2 crawls of fat past what you would've lost without the light. You are ignorant of the enhancement impact of the light on your outcomes. All you know is that you got results. You don't know how much the light added to them because it's an impact that goes on gradually over weeks and isn't something we can promptly observe or feel happening right away after the light medicines.

So much of the time, you don't generally have any method for knowing with sureness whether it is working or not simply founded on your easygoing perceptions (for example, without firmly controlling things and estimating things with versus without the light).

However, here's the uplifting news: You don't generally need to think about whether it is working because genuine science has tried these things and, as of now, demonstrated that it works! So basically, trust the science! These researchers did unquestionably more thorough and firmly controlled investigations than you would ever do in your very own understanding, so trust their work. So this means this: DO IT, and afterward, believe that you're getting valuable impacts.

Presently, there are obviously, numerous examples where one will see an impact. For instance:

- If you utilize it for relief from discomfort, you will see an immediate torment-killing impact inside 20 minutes.

- If you routinely get cut or injured here and there, and you see to what extent it usually takes you to recuperate, and afterward you do it with the light, you will see it mends a lot quicker.

- If you utilize it for balding and take photographs, you will probably see that over weeks or months, and your photos show improvement.

- If you are utilizing it for joint pain, you may see following half a month or long periods of treatment that your joints hurt much more minor and move better, or you don't get torment the day after exercise, and so on.

- If you utilize it for cellulite reduction, take photographs and watch changes over a couple of months, and you'll likely observe a noteworthy reduction.

- If you are utilizing it for wrinkle reduction and against maturing purposes, you will probably see impacts inside half a month (and may even have individuals praising you on how great you look)

In any case, once more, the critical point is that you don't need to re-think this or marvel on the off chance that it is busy because the actual controlled research has just indicated that it works. So, execute what needs to be done and realize that you are accomplishing something which science has just demonstrated works. Trust the science, and do what needs to be done!

Q: How would we be able to be sure we are duplicating the conditions in the investigations, and what precisely are the key focuses we should be aware of during our sessions?

My suggested dosing ranges in this book depend on the exploration. These general dosing rules depend on the central part of the information. So by following these dosing rules for your particular issues, you'll be by the exploration. That is all you have to know, so don't overthink it to an extreme.

Q: What are the general advantages of 660nm (red light) and 850nm (NIR) and the upsides and downsides of joining these in one unit?

As already clarified, red and close infrared act through a similar component. The significant contrast is the infiltration profundity. Be that as it may, see the past segment on red versus close infrared for a progressive nitty-gritty talk of the distinctions.

Since both red and close infrared work through similar systems, there genuinely are no all-inclusive upsides and downsides – it's subject to how you need to utilize it. If you need to use it to treat different tissues like organs, muscles, or the mind, go for unadulterated close infrared or a 50-50 blend. Red-light may be preferred if you need to be hostile to maturing or mend more in the surface tissues. In any case, if it's not too much trouble, remember that BOTH red-light and approach infrared will work for the two purposes. At the point when we talk about these distinctions, it's simply a question of degrees of adequacy, not excessively one works for a particular reason, and the other doesn't work by any means. The two of them work for basically these reasons, so don't be worried, and persuade yourself that the red light won't work for treating muscles, organs, and so forth. The one exemption maybe, where it has been demonstrated that close infrared enters much preferable through the skull over unmistakable red-light does. Then, in case you need to utilize it to improve mental wellbeing, close infrared is a superior decision,

Chapter 11: How Does Red-light Therapy Heal?

Now it is time to look at how this red light will be able to work to your benefit in helping to heal the body: Trillions of cells that make up who we are will find small structures inside of them known as "mitochondria." These are responsible for the cell's energy production in a process called "metabolism."

When a cell is given the nutrients and more than it needs to properly metabolize, a process that will involve some chemical oxidation of glucose over into carbon dioxide into the mitochondria, it is a sign that the cell is healthy doing what it is supposed to. If the breakdown of metabolism within the cells starts to happen, then this is when we begin to see more disease and cancer throughout the body.

Almost all of the primary human diseases have indeed been linked back to the mitochondrial activity in our cells. Understanding which foods and other factors can enhance metabolism and inhibit metabolism can be a lifesaver to help people prevent diseases they are already suffering from.

When you go through the process of red-light therapy, the skin will be exposed to a low-level laser. You will do this a few times a week for a specific treatment time based on your needs. You can do this indefinitely, but most people will pick to do this for a certain kind of condition, and the treatment will last for one to two months until that condition is dealt with thoroughly.

You can use a red-light therapy device from your own home if you choose, but there are also a lot of professionals who work in cosmetic clinics and other similar places that will be able to do this treatment for you as well. Either way, as long as the proper devices are being used, you will see that red-light therapy will be a great way to improve your health.

Those who believe in the power of red-light therapy believe that the low level of the laser will help kick start the body's ability to recover from a variety of conditions, diseases, and more. In addition, this laser will help the body increase the production of collagen, increase blood flow, and repair your tissues.

We need to take some time to look at the mechanics of how this kind of therapy will work. This works will be similar to what we see with other laser treatments, but the red light will work with a lower wavelength. It allows us to use it on areas that are a bit more sensitive, including the skin and the eyes, while still being safe.

When we expose the skin to light energy, it will release the adenosine - triphosphate (ATP), which is believed to help bodywork form new capillaries, boost collagen production, and repair some tissues that have been damaged.

For these reasons, there are a lot of times that people will choose to use red-light therapy to help themselves. It has been used to help treat issues in arthritis, heal burns, and smooth out stretch marks. These are just a few of the different ways you can work with the therapy, and we have discussed a few of them, along with the research that backs it up, earlier in this guidebook.

The neat thing about this is that the first FDA-approved use for this kind of therapy and the device that comes with it was used to help speed up wound healing that was going slowly. It was done because the red-light laser would penetrate the skin between 8 and 10 millimeters, absorbing it deeper into the body. Over time, when this was correctly used, it helped affect the immune system, metabolic processes, and the nervous system, to name a few.

It is essential to know how red-light therapy is different from others similar. It is all going to come down to the wavelengths of the red light. This treatment will emit some visible red light, and the lasers will be emitted at 60 nm. Some of these treatments will use more of a near-infrared light above 700 nm or below visible red light, which would be closer to 590 nm. And then, some devices are going to combine blue and red-light together. It all depends on the type of light that you decide to purchase.

When we compare this to what is seen with traditional laser therapy, we will find that these treatments will emit light at a higher density than red-light therapy. It causes more damage to the body's tissues and can cause more destruction if you are not careful. It is not a potential problem with red-light therapy because of the emitted very low-level laser.

Traditional laser therapy aims to damage the skin because it promotes body healing and revitalizes faster than without the treatment. Red-light treatment will not have enough power or heat to do this, and you don't have to worry about it burning, destroying, or injuring the body's tissues. It is seen as a more efficient method for healing than others.

It will work as some of the other laser therapies out there, in that the laser that is emitted from the light will be able to help heal the body and repair some of the cells in the body. But it will not come with any potential danger as we see with other methods, which makes it so much better to work with.

Lowering the Metabolism with Some Environmental Toxins

We need to focus on and understand when it comes to cellular metabolism that all the steps that we will work with are going to be catalyzed thanks to one specific enzyme. This enzyme is known as "cytochrome c oxidase." Dr. Otto Warburg discovered this enzyme in 1926.

So, why do we need to be able to understand this particular enzyme? This enzyme is responsible for the oxygen used by the cells in that it can interact directly with that oxygen. It will catalyze the very last step in the process of metabolism. It is essential if we want to make sure that the metabolism of the cells is going to be done correctly.

Through his research, Dr. Warburg found that we would take a previously healthy cell and then turn it cancerous when we can inhibit this enzyme. And this information has been validated through the years with other studies and experiments.

It is a huge finding that we need to spend more time on. When one enzyme is taken out, harmed, or inhibited somehow, this will be a bad thing for you. It means that the body will struggle with doing the metabolism that it needs, which causes the cell to go from one that is healthy to one that has issues and could be considered cancerous overall. According to scientists from the University of Pennsylvania in 2015,

It supports what we have been talking about all along: When the cells do not have this particular enzyme, or there is some other reason why this enzyme is not doing the work it should, there would be some issues along the way. The cells are going to deal with health conditions of all kinds, cancer, and more. Ensuring that this enzyme can work in the manner, it should and learning how to make the metabolism work properly will make a difference in the body's overall health.

A few toxins will inhibit the activity of this enzyme, including Unsaturated fatty acids, X-ray radiation, EVB radiation, serotonin, estrogen, aluminum phosphide, carbon dioxide, cyanide, chemotherapy, and more. You can control a few of these on your own if you would like, such as the fatty acids you are eating, but a few are a bit harder to control.

Let's take a look at how these are going to work: When you are exposed to any of the above contaminants of the environment, the cells are going to produce a free radical known as "nitric oxide." This free radical will bind directly to the cytochrome c oxidase that we need so desperately, and it will end up deactivating it at some point. As long as the nitric oxide stays bound to the enzyme, it means that the cell cannot metabolize in the manner it should, giving it a defective cancer metabolism in the process.

How to Enhance the Metabolism of the Cell with Some Red-light

Now, we need to look at what red-light therapy will be able to do to help us out. The impact that we will see with the near-infrared and red light on the metabolism of our cells is unique. It has spurred a lot of studies throughout the years. These lights have been shown to unbind the nitric oxide from the cytochrome c oxidase enzyme from cells.

When the red light can remove the nitric oxide, it is going to do some amazing things. The cytochrome c oxidase can get back to work, and it is going to be more energized. It helps to supercharge the enzyme's activity, speed up the metabolism there, and ensure that the cell gets back to its old healthy self rather than being diseased and even cancerous, causing trouble for you.

It is good news for you because you will see an enhancement in how the cells can metabolize again. They will get back to what they should do naturally, which has stopped them from environmental toxins. When this happens, it means that you will be able to enjoy a bunch of beneficial physiological effects that are going to emerge when the metabolic activity increases. Some of these beneficial effects include:

1. A reduction in the number of free radicals found in the cells.
2. A reduction of inflammation in the body.
3. A reduction of lactic acid that builds up in the body.
4. A reduction of stress in general.
5. An increased amount of CO_2 production.
6. An increased amount of blood will flow through the body, helping us clean out the body easier, get more energy, and improve our health overall.
7. An increased amount of cellular oxygenation.
8. An increase in the amount of energy ATP production throughout the body as well.

As you can see here, there are already a lot of health benefits that you will reap when you work with red-light therapy and other types of light therapy in the process. It will be significant because we will be able to improve with these lights allowing our bodies to heal more naturally.

We could choose to take a lot of medications to do this, but that will mask the problem and hide the symptoms rather than give us the actual relief that we want. The second we stop taking the medications is the second we are going to start feeling sick again. But with something like red-light therapy, which takes care of the condition and helps the body heal naturally, you will feel relief faster and enjoy better health in no time. And this can make a world of difference to so many people.

All these beneficial physiological options above will account for most, if not all, of the different effects that people are going to benefit from when they use near-infrared or red-light therapies to improve their health.

To summarize: infrared and red light can penetrate deeply into the tissues that are in your body. It is so important because it will help reduce the amount of nitric acid in our bodies. This healing power of removing the nitric acid and making it disappear allows the cells to finally heal and do the work they are meant to do. With just a few sessions with this light therapy, you can get relief and turn cells that could be cancerous back into healthy and happy cells again.

Chapter 12:   Methods to Use to Accelerate Your Healing with Light Therapy

Now that we know more about red-light therapy and all of the things that you can do with it, it is time to delve into some of the things you can do to see this therapy come to life and do a lot for it you.

While the red-light therapy will be decisive on its own, you will find that there are a few actions that you can take to enhance it further. These actions are often simple, but they will propel you along on this journey and make results faster and more efficient. Some of the steps that you can use to get the most out of the red-light therapy include:

Do Two Sessions a Day

You can certainly choose to work with one session a day if you would like, but often, people find that they will get the most out of their treatment when they can do two or even three sessions during the day. The trick here is to experiment and see what is going to work the best for you.

When you choose to do light therapy more than once a day, you heal the cells and keep all of that nitric acid out of the body. And you are going to be amazed at the difference this makes. You will feel like there is more energy inside of you when it is time to start the morning, and it can be an excellent way to turn the body down after a long day of working and putting aside all of your other obligations for the day.

Of course, if you find that only one treatment can do the work you need or find it challenging to fit the sessions in more than once, it is acceptable to stick with that number of sessions for your needs. But many patients who use this therapy and see the best results will like working with the red-light at least a few times a day.

Get Plenty of Sleep

The next thing that we need to focus on here is the idea of getting yourself plenty of sleep regularly. When you are short on sleep, you are not giving your body the time that it needs to replenish itself or clean out some of the toxins that plague it. Even if you are working with the red-light therapy, if you are not taking in enough sleep regularly, the body will not be able to clear itself out, and you will not feel better.

But getting enough sleep can be a struggle for many people. Learning how to take care of yourself, get off the phone, and reduce your stress levels is all necessary if you want to sleep at night. But some of the things that you can do to help you get to sleep fast and stay asleep all night includes:

1. Keep work at work: If you often bring your work home with you, it will be hard for you to learn how to get to bed on time. This kind of lifestyle usually means that you are stressed and won't turn your mind off when you go to bed.

2. Turn off electronics before bed: If possible, turn off all electronics about an hour before going to bed. It helps detoxify the brain from the light emitted from the computer, phone, and more to relax. Consider reading, writing, or starting your bedtime routine during this time instead.

3. Make a list of the things you need to do the next day: It is hard to get to sleep at night if you have a million thoughts and things to remember running through your brain. Before you head to bed, please make a list of the items you want to get done so you no longer have to worry about remembering them later.

4. Be more active during the day: It may be hard to keep up your activity levels if you are sitting at a desk all day or not to do much. Instead of letting that happen, you need to find ways to be more active so that your brain is ready to go to sleep. Whether that means getting up and moving more or starting a workout routine, you have to find the method of activity that works the best for you.

5. Start a nighttime routine: It is an excellent way to tell your brain that it is time to turn off and go to bed. Starting this a while before you hit the hay will make a world of difference as well. You can make it as long, as short, as easy, or as complicated as you would like. Just stick with the same routine each day.

6. Turn off the lights: Sleeping in the dark is usually the best. You will find that this helps signal to the brain that it is time to go to sleep. Find any of the lights in the room that may be keeping you awake at night and figure out how to turn them off or get rid of them.

7. No television in the bedroom: Many people like to fall asleep with a TV in their room. They think that this helps them to fall asleep at night. While you may be able to get to sleep with the noise and the light of the television going, your rest is not going to be very deep. Please turn it off or get it out of the room and see what a difference it can make for you.

8. Listen to some quiet and soft music if needed: Some people find that the noises outside their windows are too loud or have trouble with the quiet. If this is the case for you, do not let it be an excuse to go out and grab the television. Instead, turn on some soft classical music or some music to the sounds of nature, and let that be what helps to lull you to sleep at night.

Getting enough sleep will be critical if you want to see the benefits of red-light therapy. It is hard to do this, but putting yourself first and learning when to say no to other obligations and temptations can help make it a bit easier.

Eat Lots of Healthy Foods

To help your cells function well, and if you want to get the most out of the red-light therapy, you need to be more aware of your consuming foods. You do not want to do the red-light therapy and then go fill up on brownies and ice cream the whole time. Instead, filling the body up with healthy foods and will give the body the nutrition it needs to get healthier and do the necessary repairs is going to be critical.

It brings up the question of how you are supposed to eat healthily.

You do not need to follow a strict diet or go on something hard to follow. If you want to lose more weight while doing the treatment, that is fine, but eating foods that are good for you and made with real ingredients rather than processed ingredients will see better results.

So, to make sure that you are eating foods that will help fill you up and ensure that you are getting the nutrition you need, think about foods in their natural states. Eating lots of fresh fruits and vegetables, lean meat and protein sources, healthy cooking oils, good dairy products with no added sugars, and whole-grain carbohydrates will do the trick. Learn how to do the correct portion sizes and listen to your body when it is hungry or not, and you will start to see results in your health as well.

Learn How to Get Rid of the Junk

While it may be fine to have a bit of junk food on occasion when you crave something sweet, most of us enjoy way too many sweets and junk food that we do not need. We take in lots of carbohydrates, sugars, baked goods, sodas and juices, and so much more. And this ends up being bad for us overall.

If you want to reduce the problems that you have with your cells and many diseases, you need to help the red-light treatment out a bit by cutting out some of the junk. Limit yourself to just a bit of those on occasion, rather than making it a staple in your diet plan. It can be challenging, and you may need to go through a bit of detoxification to make it happen. But if you can stick with this, you will see some significant changes in your health.

Drink Lots of Water

You will want to make sure that you are getting all of the toxins out of your body during this treatment while staying hydrated and making sure that your organs and all parts of your body will work well. Too often, we are too busy with our days or be drinking coffee, pop, and other drinks, and we do not make sure that we will give the body the optimal hydration that we need from the water.

It should be your goal to take in a minimum of eight to ten glasses of water a day. If you are still thirsty after that, do exercise, or deal with a scorching day, then try to drink more. It will help you get as much out of the red-light therapy as possible, and even a little bit of extra water in your day will be enough to help you feel better too.

Conclusion

We have looked at everything to know about red-light therapy; how it works, the benefits, how to go about red-light therapy, including choosing the correct device and dosage, and the tips to keep in mind in terms of treatment guidelines.

Keep in mind that red-light therapy and all his forms are still alternatives. It means unless advised so by a qualified professional, you should avoid any situation that calls on you to use red-light therapy as the only way to manage a more profound condition. As we mentioned severally throughout this book, red-light therapy seems to work well when coupled with other wellbeing strategies.

If you decide that the benefits are well worth it, check with your dermatologist or physician, which could be the best treatment and device for your situation.

You should safely use red-light and derive the many tangible benefits we discussed in earlier parts of this book.